Clinical Trials and the African Person

Value Inquiry Book Series

VOLUME 319

African American Philosophy

Edited by

J. Everet Green, *Mercy College*
John H. McClendon III, *Michigan State University*

The titles published in this series are listed at *brill.com/vibs* and *brill.com/afam*

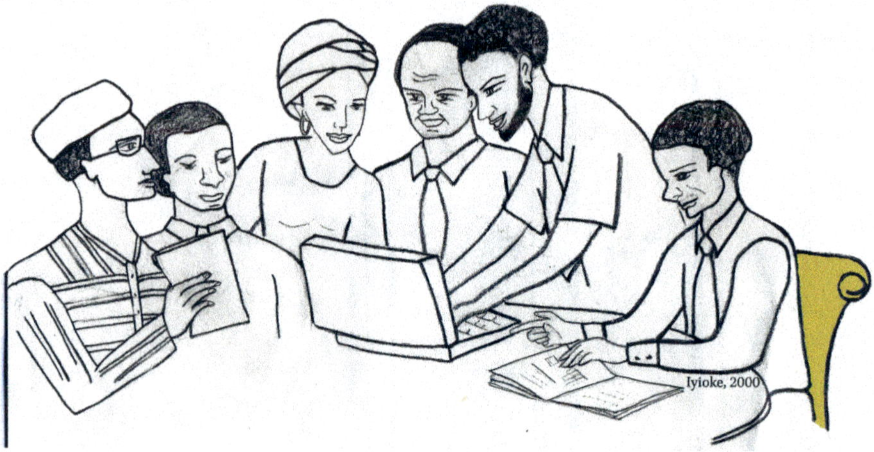

"Whatever happens to the individual happens to the family or community in which he belongs. Likewise, the African disposition sees health topics (wellbeing or illness) as a communal affair, sometimes to the point that family or community has a stake in becoming aware of another's health condition and having a role in the decisions regarding his treatment."
FIGURE BY THE AUTHOR

Clinical Trials and the African Person

A Quest to Re-Conceptualize Responsibility

By

Ike Valentine Iyioke

BRILL
RODOPI

LEIDEN | BOSTON

Library of Congress Cataloging-in-Publication Data

Names: Iyioke, Ike V., author.
Title: Clinical trials and the African person : a quest to re-conceptualize responsibility / by Ike Valentine Iyioke.
Description: Leiden ; Boston : Brill-Rodopi, 2018. | Series: Value inquiry book series, ISSN 0929-8436 ; volume 319. African American philosophy | Includes bibliographical references and index.
Identifiers: LCCN 2018016455 (print) | LCCN 2018017649 (ebook) | ISBN 9789004366947 (E-book) | ISBN 9789004366602 (pbk. : alk. paper)
Subjects: LCSH: Medical ethics. | African Americans--Medical care. | Public health--Moral and ethical aspects--Cross-cultural studies.
Classification: LCC R724 (ebook) | LCC R724 .I95 2018 (print) | DDC 174.2089/96073--dc23
LC record available at https://lccn.loc.gov/2018016455

Typeface for the Latin, Greek, and Cyrillic scripts: "Brill". See and download: brill.com/brill-typeface.

ISSN 0929-8436
ISBN 978-90-04-36660-2 (paperback)
ISBN 978-90-04-36694-7 (e-book)

This book is printed on acid-free paper and produced in a sustainable manner.

I dedicate this book to the Iyioke family: first, to my dear wife Ifeoma Chika Iyioke, PhD., our sons IkeNna Jr. [10], ArinzeChukwu [7], IliloChi [5], and daughter SopuruChi [3 months!]; whose moral and material support (plus emotional 'harassment') have made my experience at Michigan State University a life-long lesson to cherish. It is in them that I find my anchor.

Above all, I owe everything to God Almighty who is ever faithful even in my unfaithfulness.

We are who we are because of where we belong.

IKE IYIOKE

Contents

PART 2
Responsibility

PART 3
Personhood

Preface

This book is an attempt to explore the ethics of public health, specifically, ethical issues with clinical trials; it is also a reflection of the wider area, and research forays that I make in the field of bioethics. In it, I aim to re-conceptualize responsibility in clinical trials with the insight of the African notion of self. I strive to complement scholarly literature dealing with cross-cultural biomedical ethics, and emphasize the African perspective which is rare or even non-existent in some cases.

To take on this task of reconceptualization first, I recognize that bioethics as a field has continued to spread out from its American birthplace to numerous cultural milieus across the globe. Accompanying this spread is the challenge of how to integrate and apply its founding principles. Faster still is the pace at which the Global South has become the choice site for a sizeable chunk of the clinical trial enterprise from the Global North.

Of the many problems with principlism, the one that is most directly antithetical to my thesis is its excessive individualist emphasis, focusing on individual rights, his autonomy, etc., to the detriment of everything else. In so doing, much is left to be desired. Hence, its numerous revisions even in Western practice of research ethics clearly point to some inbred difficulties in its application. That, in and of itself, further buoys my argument for a robust alternative – an African perspective (a communalist set of principles, presented here as bio-eco-communalism or BEC).

Further still, it has become obvious that the assumptions implicit in the Western framework that makes claim to universal validity are not shared by non-Western cultures. If not reined in, the concern seems to be that the Euro-American approach is bound to globalize a less than global view of the world and reality. In other words, the mainstream research ethics which is grounded on principlism is itself inherently linked to Western individualistic notions of personhood, whereas the rest of the world, particularly Africa, sees the person not as an isolated individual, but as a part of the community who is embedded in kinship, group, community and the environment. Likewise, many authors have noted that the totality of the African world-view in which the people's ethics is rooted, and the societal activities which center on the promotion of vitality and fertility of human beings, livestock, and the land on which their livelihood depends, are entirely missed by principlism.

In the face of this, I urge for a reappraisal of sorts about the place of responsibility for human subjects in research. More specifically, as many clinical trials are off-shored abroad, it provides an opportunity to weigh in on the Western emphasis on individualism and to acknowledge the cultural systems of other peoples, for instance, communitarianism (or communalism). While opposing individualism (a Euro-American mantra), the African perspective stresses communitarianism. By definition, the communitarianist philosophical view point instantly recognizes that ethical issues with biomedical studies are far more broad-based.

Therefore, responsibility in clinical trials *must* in tandem, be broad-based. There is no debate that research studies do impact the individual person, but that impact extends in varying degrees to everyone and everything else around him/her – family, neighborhood, community and even the physical environment. Put otherwise, responsibility in biomedical studies particularly, those dealing with human subjects (and in bioethics as a whole), must be seen to extend beyond the individual person and to encompass the community and the physical environment within which the individual resides. Because the African notion of selfhood is communalist and broad-based, it is adequately structured to address the short-comings in the mainstream individualist perspective. As such, responsibility for (and by) the individual can only make sense through the community in which he/she is rooted. Consequently, I urge that the current understanding of responsibility be re-conceptualized. When this is done, responsibility for human subjects in research (particularly in adequately suited cultural environments), will henceforth mean responsibility for the individual rights, plus, those of his family, community, and the ecosystem.

Acknowledgements

The following people provided invaluable inputs to this work: Dr. Ann Mongoven was very supportive particularly assisting with skill acquisition in bioethics practice (for instance, serving as my practicum mentor and providing referrals for my IRB membership accreditation). Dr. Jim Roper was invaluable in so many ways, for instance, his knack for giving criticisms in the most humane and painless manner is remarkable. He often reassured me that I could disagree with his views [and he *meant* it].

Dr. Paul Thompson bequeathed to me more published materials than I can count; not least of them is what I've called, the "Manna from Paul" – *Guidance Framework for Testing of Genetically Modified Mosquitoes* for my Chapter 2. It has been the icing on the cake. And for Dr. John McClendon III – what do you call someone who rectified your doctoral admission process; saw you through the thick and thin of the program, up until the very end – father figure? That's what he is, and much more.

Next, my deep gratitude is also due to my big sister Mrs. Ifeyinwa Mary Agnes Ugwuoke, BA, MA, LLB, LLM. Her outpouring of 'libations' to God Almighty in faraway homeland (Nigeria), has had profound positive effect on my family in the New World (USA). Finally, the author would like to thank J. Everet Green, PhD., for his input on earlier drafts of this book; as well as other anonymous reviewers for their comments.

List of Illustrations

List of Abbreviations/Terms

Adverse Drug Reaction (ADR)	A response to a drug that is noxious and unintended and occurs at doses normally used in a person for the prophylaxis, diagnosis or therapy of disease, or for modification of physiological function. Adverse drug reactions are classified into six types (with mnemonics): dose-related (Augmented), non-dose-related (Bizarre), dose-related and time-related (Chronic), time-related (Delayed), withdrawal (End of use), and failure of therapy (Failure).
Adverse Event (AE)	Any untoward medical occurrence in a patient or clinical investigation subject to whom a pharmaceutical product is administered. An AE can therefore be any unfavorable and unintended sign (including an abnormal laboratory finding), symptom, or disease temporally associated with the use of a medicinal (investigational) product, whether or not related to the medicinal (investigational) product.
All-in-one (one-in-all)	A term I have coined to depict the suffusion and inseparability of the individual into his or her community and environment.
Alleles	Different forms of the same gene, usually arising through mutation, that are responsible for hereditary variation.
BEC	Bio-eco-communalism just like the concept of one-in-all, refers to the inseparability of the individual within his/her community and environment.
Biome	A term from the Greek *bios*, meaning relation to life; used in ecology to include major life in the area, such as tundra biome, tropical rainforest biome and grassland biome.
Biomass	The amount of matter of biological origin in a given area, for example, the living and decaying matter in the soil, as opposed to the inorganic mineral components such as sand, silt and clay.
Biosphere	(a) The zone on the earth's surface where all life exists; (b) all living organisms of the earth.

Biota	All species of plants and animals occurring in a specific area.
CRS	Corporate social responsibility is a duty or an inbuilt commitment by corporate bodies to uphold ethical values and ensure quality of life of the workforce, the local community and the physical environment, while earning profits.
Ecosystem	A biological system composed of a community of organisms and the nonliving environment with which it interacts [same for Environment and Ecology].
GMM	Genetically Modified Mosquitoes, also called genetically engineered mosquitoes, transgenic mosquitoes, or living modified mosquitoes – mosquitoes that have heritable traits derived through use of recombinant DNA technology, which alter the strain, line, or colony in a manner usually intended to result in reduction of the transmission of mosquito – borne human diseases.[1]
The Global North[2]	Also known as the industrialized world, Western, or Euro-American – refers to the 57 countries with high human development that have a Human Development Index above .8 as reported in the United Nations Development Program Report 2005. Most, but not all, of these countries are located in the Northern Hemisphere.
Global South[3]	The industrializing world or The Global South refers to the countries of the rest of the world, most of which are located in the Southern Hemisphere. It includes both countries with medium human development index, HDI (88 countries with an HDI less than .8 and greater than .5) and low human development index (32 countries with an HDI of less than .5). Thus defined, the Global South is made up of some 133 countries out of a total of 197. Most

1 This is one of few definitions derived from the WHO GMM project (see Chapter 2).

2 Harold Damerow, http://faculty.ucc.edu/egh-damerow/global_south.htm. Viewed on February 25, 2015.

3 Ibid.

	of the Global South is located in South and Central America, Africa, and Asia.
Holism	The interconnectivity and interdependence of all things in reality.
Serious Adverse Event, SAE, or Serious Adverse Drug Reaction, Serious ADR	Any untoward medical occurrence that at any dose results in death, is life-threatening, requires inpatient hospitalization or prolongation of existing hospitalization, results in persistent or significant disability/incapacity, or is a congenital anomaly/birth defect.
Vulnerable subjects	Individuals whose willingness to volunteer in a clinical trial may be unduly influenced by the expectation, whether justified or not, of benefits associated with participation, or of a retaliatory response from senior members of a hierarchy in case of refusal to participate. Examples are members of a group with a hierarchical structure, such as medical, pharmacy, dental, and nursing students, subordinate hospital and laboratory personnel, employees of the pharmaceutical industry, members of the armed forces, and persons kept in detention. Other vulnerable subjects include patients with incurable diseases, persons in nursing homes, unemployed or impoverished persons, patients in emergency situations, ethnic minority groups, homeless persons, nomads, refugees, minors, pregnant women, and those incapable of giving consent.

Introduction

Advances in biomedical research epitomize the dizzying strides in modern science. These quintessential feats, thanks to clinical trials, represent the unleashing of the human brain power in making dreams a reality by improving mankind's physical, emotional, and material conditions. However, scientific research has sometimes become more a search for material gains, absolute control and might; and less a science in quest of the truth. When science fashions a project to serve such agendas, the avowed purpose of dominating nature can easily turn into the domination of the human person,[1] and ethical problems of enormous proportions often do arise; problems to which science has no clue, much less an answer. Hence, the very essence of humanity stands the risk of being compromised, sometimes irreversibly.[2]

While science cannot advance without experimentation, pursuit of narrow scientific goals and populist economic motives have sometimes led to troubling behaviors by some scientists which undermine research ethics guidelines and principles. And as Western[3] research arenas continue to tighten their regulatory noose, coupled with the rapidly drying pool of volunteer enrollees,[4] some researchers are compelled to seek out 'soft targets' elsewhere, including Africa; after all, water always follows the path of least resistance.

As the Global South becomes the choice site for a sizeable chunk of the clinical trials enterprise, in this book I urge for a reappraisal of sorts, and for a harder scrutiny about the place of responsibility in clinical trials. My thesis is to reformulate the concept of responsibility by replacing the notion of personhood via principlism lenses with the concept of personhood from a communalist perspective. Question: should science be left to push its empiricist/materialist agenda unchecked? More specifically, as clinical trials continue to settle into new locales across the world including the Global South, it seems about time to halt the Western extreme emphasis on individualism and the tendency to fuse, at all costs, knowledge and might, and truly acknowledge other philosophical

1 Person, man, self, individual, human being/person, and to a lesser extent, identity, have been used interchangeably in this book to mean the same thing (in line with existing literary corpus). However, there are places where exceptions may be made.

2 Okere, Theophilus. 2005. *Philosophy, Culture, and Society in Africa.* Nsukka: Afro-Orbis Publications Ltd., p. 153.

3 Western, Euro-American, the Global North, the industrialized world, all mean the same thing in this work. On the other hand, the Global South, the industrializing world, the emerging economies, Africa, etc., all refer to the same region.

4 Find an exhaustive discussion on this in Adriana Petryna's *When Experiments Travel* (2009).

 | DOI 10.1163/9789004366947_002

and cultural systems. The central argument is that we must recalibrate responsibility around the following question: is the autonomy-based principlism still relevant in research ethics as compared to the communalist perspective (for whose benefit and at whose expense)?

It has been made apparent that the assumptions implicit in the framework that makes claim to universal validity are not shared by non-western cultures.[5] If not reined in, the concern seems to be that the approach is bound to "globalize a less than global view of the world and reality."[6] For instance, the mainstream research ethics purports to adhere to the principlist quartet,[7] which is inherently linked to Western individualistic notions of personhood, whereas much of the rest of the world, including Africa, sees the person not as an isolated individual, but as a part of the community who is embedded in kinship, group and community. Also, while the African concept of a person is unitary, the Euro-American concept is essentially split between persons and non-persons within the human species. For instance, fetuses, human infants, young children, people with mental disorder, and patients in persistent vegetative state may be technically considered as non-persons because they do not possess any moral standing in the secular moral community. Tristram Engelhardt makes this strident point in *The Foundations of Bioethics,* a polemic publication that has significantly shaped today's mainstream bioethical practice. Moreover, a slew of other considerations is entirely missed by these principles. They include, the holism of the African world-view in which the people's ethics is rooted; and the societal activities which center on the promotion of vitality and fertility of human beings, livestock, and the land on which their livelihood depends. African philosophical concepts are never considered as individuated concepts, rather they are holistic. Hence, it is rife to see how an ethical discussion can morph into and encompass religious, metaphysical, ontological, social or cultural spheres.

This book presents a tripartite thesis: responsibility, clinical trials, and personhood (specifically, the African notion of personhood). The challenge is to

---

5 See Chikezie Onuoha's analysis of *Bioethics Without Borders: An African Perspective*. An unpublished doctoral dissertation, Uppsala University, Uppsala, Sweden, 2007.

6 Confer Widdows, H. 2007. "Is Global Ethics Moral Neo-colonialism? An Investigation of the Issue in the Context of Bioethics." *Bioethics*, 21, 6: 305–315; 2007. Other commentators, just like Okere (2005: 154), have argued similarly.

7 The four principles of bioethics (a.k.a., principlism) for mainstream bioethics are: respect for autonomy (a norm of respecting the decision-making capacities of autonomous persons); non-maleficence (a norm of avoiding the causation of harm); beneficence (a group of norms for providing benefits and balancing benefits against risks and costs); and, justice (a group of norms for distributing benefits, risks, and costs fairly).

harmoniously blend these seemingly disparate themes (full-fledge concepts in their own rights), to justify why it makes sense to couple them together for my purpose. On another front, it is easy to misconstrue my reference to 'African notion of personhood,' as essentializing. As I shall prove, particularly in Chapter 4, I am not overgeneralizing. In fact, beneath the apparent diversity of African philosophical expressions of the self, there is a fundamental and undisputed uniformity, thus setting the stage for a clear-cut cultural relativity (ethical particularism). As with many other African concepts, something that Egbeke Aja's 2006 work attests to, values seem to vary from one society to another, but under a close scrutiny, "in terms of their functions and interrelationships, some general principles emerge." Abundant literature backs up the fact that this is most prevalent in Black Africa; and similarities to these abound in much of North ('Arab') Africa as well.

Part 1 is composed of Chapters 1 and 2 which discuss respective sides (each in contra-opposition) of clinical trials that are germane to my exegesis. The 'clinical trials' theme – both as the fulcrum of research ethics and as a concept – has endured since the dawn of experimentation, presenting a platform for analyses on a wide range of issues. That platform is pivotal (if not more so) today than it has ever been. After some preliminaries, Chapter 1 looks at the historical trend that foreshadowed modern biomedical research and ends with the Nigeria-Pfizer Trovan case study. The big pharma experiment in Nigeria stands as a forefront warning that bad practices have been breaking loose on a neo-colonial model. The 1996 clinical trials which followed severe meningitis and cholera outbreaks in a northern Nigerian city that involved huge ethical issues with the American pharmaceutical giant Pfizer, provide both the catalyst and a test case for this book.

Chapter 2 reviews relevant aspects of the WHO-sponsored *Guidance Framework for Testing of Genetically Modified Mosquitoes,* by highlighting the excellent and easily replicable examples it has set for clinical trial procedures. In sum, it prescribes remedies that could be used to fix all the glaring deficiencies attributable in a case like the Pfizer's Trovan.

Part 2 – Chapter 3, deliberates on the concept of responsibility. Ordinarily, 'responsibility' is a conceptual theme some theorists claim to have long analyzed and reduced to smithereens. In this book, I don't have to reinvent the wheel, but I make bold to present what could pass as an unorthodox but valid perspective of the concept.

Finally, Part 3 – Chapter 4, examines personhood from an African perspective and hones in on my conclusions. Personhood is introduced as a third panel to the equilibrium by bringing to bear its African philosophical dimensions. I wish to use the notion of personhood in African thought to provide a perspective of what responsibility can mean in an African context and then apply it to biomedical clinical trials with human subjects. Ultimately, the African philosophical notion of selfhood will put in perspective my argument to re-conceptualize responsibility in clinical trials. More specifically, while opposing individualism (a Euro-American mantra), the African perspective stresses communalism/communitarianism. As such, responsibility for (and by) the individual can only make sense through the community in which he/she is rooted. Ultimately, the themes of responsibility, clinical trials, and the African concept of personhood, come to a full circle.

PART 1

Clinical Trials

CHAPTER 1

Who is Responsible for Human Subjects (When Experiments Travel)?

1.1 Introduction

The question that this chapter seeks to answer – as shown in the title – is not new. In fact, it is so old it is now trite and rhetorical. However, the upshot is that it needs to be re-contextualized, and then answered. I would thus address it in the context of a new dispensation – a globalized clinical trials dispensation.

In the current globalized world, it is daunting to keep track of the tremendous amount of clinical trial projects that are ongoing at any one time. As such, a few of the questions that dogged us in the wake of landmark clinical trial abuses including the ones by the Nazi doctors in concentration camps have both lingered on as well as become more complicated. The atrocities led to the Nuremberg code of 1947, a direct result of Nuremberg War Crime Trials after WWII. It set standards for judging physicians and scientists who conduct biomedical experiments to guarantee that research involving human subjects are carried out in an ethically accepted manner. As I will shortly review, other codes and guidelines that have emerged include the Helsinki Declaration (of 1964, but which has been revised numerous times); the 1974 U.S. Code of Federal Regulations (45 CFR Part 46); and the 1979 Belmont Report of the U.S. National Commission; all of which outline ethical principles and guidelines for the protection of human subjects of biomedical, social and behavioral research. The challenge still is how to end abusive research and promote quality ones that protect research subjects *everywhere*. Hence, the following questions remain pertinent: How should human research subjects be protected? Who should provide them protection? In our increasingly interconnected world, how can we ensure compliance, guideline consistency, and checks and balances across borders? These questions remain relevant particularly because even as most clinical studies today are initiated and registered in the Global North (predominantly in the U.S.), the actual trials are sometimes outsourced and offshored[1] (often to the Global South).

1 Refer to Adriana Petryna's *When Experiments Travel* (2009), p. 2ff. Also, confer the *U.S. National Institutes of Health*, "Trends, Charts, and Maps," at, http://clinicaltrials.gov/ct2/resources/trends#RegisteredStudiesOverTimePostedResults. Viewed on October 11, 2013.

 | DOI 10.1163/9789004366947_003

The 2001 Presidential Ethics Advisory Board Report suggests two principal approaches to improving the protections of human participants in international clinical trials. (1) Relying on reviews by U.S. IRBs and assurance processes to supplement and enhance local measures or determining that a host country or host country institution has a system of protections at least equivalent to that of the United States. And, (2) helping host countries build the capacity to independently conduct clinical trials and to carry out their own scientific and ethical review. But sadly enough, these idealities emerge from flawed moral and epistemological assumptions.

Coupled with the changing geography is the fact that private sector research by, for example, pharmaceutical companies have led the way since the 1980s. And foremost in their approach is speed and profitability.[2] That approach is a concern that triggers further questions: If they are so disposed, would responsibility for study subjects be paramount on their minds? Even so, would they additionally be bound by the local systems (socio-cultural, political, and legal systems where available) and/or would they abide only by international codes of research conduct as though they were in their home countries (where enforcements are strict)? It has forcefully been argued that the financial interest and overwhelming corporate influence in test results by companies, unduly influence the drug testing system. It is therefore the in-built bias that distorts the accuracy and acceptability of drug research.[3]

The core questions of, how should human research subjects be protected; who should protect them; and how can we ensure compliance and guideline consistency across borders, directly link up with the overarching claim in this book for the need to re-conceive responsibility in clinical trials. As I will make apparent, it is by redefining 'responsibility' that we rejig our understanding in the context of an increasingly globalized world, including complexities associated with cultural, social, and political realities. The burden of my argument will be to demonstrate that this recommendation is a crying urgency if we must truly reflect the meaning of our moral condition in the field of biomedical research.

This chapter is divided into four main parts. I will start by sketching out an overview of the historical background to human experimentation in biomedicine. Next, I will review some of the U.S. and international research ethics guidelines which resulted from the events that preceded them. The intent is

2 Ibid, p. 12.

3 Shapiro, Sydney. 1978. "Divorcing Profit Motivation from New Drug Research: A Consideration of Proposals to Provide the FDA with Reliable Test Data." *Duke Law Journal*, Ninth Annual Administrative Law Issue, p. 155.

to revisit and re-reflect on provisions they have for protecting human study subjects. Third, I will briefly examine the concomitant implications of outsourcing of biomedical research to the Global South. Fourth – and for serving as the inspiration for this book – I will introduce the Pfizer-Nigeria (Trovan) case study for illustration and analysis.

1.2 Experimentation with Human Subjects: A Selective Rehash

The aphorism, "First, do no harm," is a marquee nameplate often attributed to Hippocrates.[4] It also is one that probably traces the historical explanation for why the individual's innate value – either as a patient or a patient-subject – is always of preeminent consideration in healthcare settings. Thereafter, the principal ethic of Western medicine (and later much of non-Western world) profess it as part of the Hippocratic Oath "which sets forth an array of ethical norms and functions as the pledge of the medical profession to uphold ethical standards of care."[5]

The understanding at the time was that the Hippocratics routinely 'experimented'[6] – from the Latin root *experimentum*, meaning, making a proof or trying out – with patients particularly because doctor-patient interaction always meant some sort of testing out or discovering the unknown,

> Any encounter between a doctor and a patient can be experiential and thus experimental, if only in a passing sense. The Hippocratics, who were interested in the rhythms and natural histories of disease, and in carefully observing sick people, were increasing their own experience. Further, any therapeutic innovation, even if the doctor believed it to be in the patient's interest, was an experiment.[7]

4 It has however been demonstrated that the Hippocratics of the third and fourth centuries BC actually crafted that phrase from interpreting and propagating Hippocrates' writings, including *Epidemics*, Bk. 1, Sect. XI. For more, see Carl Coleman, et al.'s (2005) *The Ethics and Regulation of Research with Human Subjects*, New Jersey: Matthew Bender and Company, Inc., p. 3. See also, "Oath of Hippocrates," in *Hippocratic Writings* (translated by J.C. Chadwick and W.N. Man, 1950).

5 Ibid, p. 3.

6 As opposed to the contemporary meaning, 'experimenting' mostly meant 'experiencing.'

7 Bynum, William. 1988. "Reflections on the History of Human Experimentation." *The Use of Human Beings in Research*. Spicker, Stuart et al, eds., 32.

In addition, the Hippocratics sometimes treated the socially and economically disadvantaged public as motivated by *philanthropia* (love of man) and *philotechnia* (love of the art [of healing]). The art of healing also included the quest to expand scientific knowledge and as such encompassed experimentation with new procedures and drugs.[8] Most of the human subjects were prisoners and condemned criminals.

The Medieval era that followed witnessed a health care delivery system that differed markedly between the rich and the poor. And just as it is today, religious moralists and ethicists of the time not only defined and crystalized the need for moral responsibilities, they also pilloried the tendency to use the poor (and other vulnerable populations) for experimentation.[9] This was happening as testing for new drugs and medical procedures were gaining currency. Experiments were also sometimes conducted on other human subjects like friends and neighbors; and curiously, on physicians themselves and their family members; and, on animal models. Commonly called 'the hierarchy of drug testing,' this practice went from domesticated non-human animals such as birds and brutes, to hospital patients and to a group that was then called the 'lesser brethren' (e.g., persons with disability and inmates of mental institutions), and so on.[10]

David Rothman recounts further as follows.

> Legends tell of ancient and medieval rulers who tested the efficacy of poison po[r]tions on condemned prisoners and released those who survived. Much better documented is the example of Lady Mary Wortley Montagu, wife of the British ambassador to Turkey, who learned about Turkish success in inoculating patients with small amounts of the smallpox material to provide immunity. Eager to convince English physicians to adopt the procedure, she persuaded King George I to run the trial by pardoning any condemned inmate at the Newgate Prison who agreed to the inoculation. In August 1721, six volunteers were inoculated; they developed local lesions but no serious illness, and all were released.[11]

8 Ibid, pp. 32–33.

9 Amundsen, Darrel. 1981. "Casuistry and Professional Obligations: The Regulation of Physicians by the Court of Conscience in the Middle Ages." *Transactions and Studies of the College Physicians of Philadelphia*, Part 1, in Series 5, 3, 22:34–35.

10 Bynum, p. 34.

11 Rothman, David. 2003. *Strangers at the Bedside: A History of How Law and Bioethics Transformed Medical Decision Making.* New York: Aldine de Gruyter, p. 21.

1.2.1 *Burroughs Wellcome (Now GlaxoSmithKline) Experiments*

Fast forward to a 20th century biomedical experimentation. In June 2014, a hot-off-the-press news flash by the British paper, *Daily Mail*,[12] divulged the discovery of a macabre mass grave of about 800 infants who were victims of diphtheria vaccine trials [in Irish Republic and the U.K.]. Historian Catherine Corless and Professor Michael Dwyer's study of death records first revealed that 2,051 children and babies in several Irish 'mother and baby' care homes were used as guinea pigs by the international drug giant Burroughs Wellcome (now GlaxoSmithKline) between 1930 and 1936. Though shocking as it is, this revelation was only but a hint of a much bizarre issue the total size of which was much greater. More bewildering still was that no record of these experimentations could be traced to the local government and public health departments, the municipal health reports, or the company's archives in London. One can only assume that this style of vaccine trials was frowned upon and rejected by the Irish government at all levels as well as the public. But on the flip side, "the fact that reports of these trials were published in the most prestigious medical journals suggests that this type of human experimentation was largely accepted by medical practitioners and facilitated by authorities in charge of children's residential institutions."[13]

While a good number of the early experiments with human subjects took place in Europe and elsewhere, the American medical environment was not immune to the practice. In fact, some of the most egregious episodes in the last century, for instance, have happened on the American soil.[14] Here, I randomly revisit (with trepidation) a few examples that took place in the U.S. (and sometimes jointly in Europe). This intentional move is aimed to highlight how each of the events presented a critical piece of lesson in the history of biomedical research.

---

12 Harriet Arkell and Neil Michael, *Daily Mail*, http://www.dailymail.co.uk/news/article-2650475/More-mass-baby-graves-Ireland-Prime-Minister-Enda-Kenny-orders-investigation-memorial-800-dead-babies-planned.html. Viewed on June 6, 2014.

13 Ibid.

14 More detailed historical narratives and the American judicial reaction to crimes committed in the guise of medical research using human subjects can be found in David Rothman's (2003) *Strangers at the Bedside* and Carl Colman, et al.'s (2005) *The Ethics and Regulation of Research with Human Subjects*, New Jersey: Matthew Bender and Company, Inc. Also, get more of the "Report of Robert H. Jackson to the President," Department of State Bulletin, at http://www.ibiblio.org/pha/war.term/trib_07.html. Viewed on May 13, 2014.

1.2.2 *Tuskegee Syphilis Study (1932–1972)*

The share size, the length of time, the bleating racial intent, and the funding source, all make this study stand out like a sore thumb. In all, 600 poor black sharecroppers (399 with latent syphilis infection, 201 without the disease) were harvested from rural Macon County, Alabama into the Tuskegee Syphilis Study. For about 40 years the subjects were denied any genuine treatment and corned to believe they were being treated for a blood disorder condition or 'bad blood,' but in actuality it was done merely to compile "data on the effects of the spontaneous evolution of syphilis on black males."[15] In return, the subjects got free food, basic stipends, medical care and burial insurance. The outing of this study in the *New York Times*, detailed it as the "the longest nontherapeutic experiment on human beings in medical history";[16] a fact that was made even worse by the revelation that indeed the U.S. government bankrolled it.

On May 16, 1997, and at the invitation of six surviving study subjects and some relatives of other families, President Bill Clinton tendered a state apology declaring his heart-felt *mea culpa* on behalf of a "government which orchestrated a study so clearly racist." He signaled it can never be allowed to happen again. The despicable act stands in contrast with everything the country, a self-styled leader of the free world, stands for and which it must stand against.[17]

1.2.3 *Nuremberg Experiments*

The superlative headliner of all biomedical experimental atrocities involving humans were perhaps the set of medical experiments in concentration camps mainly during World War II and the Holocaust in the early 1940s. As is now common knowledge, the atrocities were committed by Nazi German doctors on war victims including children of Jewish, Polish, Russian and Roman (Gypsy) origins, but had, and continues to have a worldwide impact. The crimes resulted in the prosecution of the perpetrators as war criminals before the Nuremberg military tribunal. American judges oversaw the legal proceedings during which 16 of the physicians were found guilty; seven were sentenced to death and executed on June 1948.[18]

15 Ibid, p. 42.

16 Ibid, p. 41.

17 "Apology for study done in Tuskegee" The White House Office of the Press Secretary. 1997.

18 Refer to Carl Colman et al, pp. 16–17. Contrast this with the Tuskegee experiment which got only state apology after decades of protestations. No one was either prosecuted or executed. The "Black Lives Matter" movement could have roots in events like this.

1.2.4 *Radiation Experiments*

The 1940s and the 1950s were replete with surreptitious U.S. government-sponsored experiments conducted on hospital patients and other human subjects for the testing of radiation mostly for military purposes due to the Cold War. In the words of Coleman, et al.:

> Between 1944 and 1974, the federal government funded a series of radiation experiments, including the injection of plutonium into unsuspecting hospital patients as well as the intentional release of radiation into the environment for research purposes. Some were conducted to advance biomedical science, while others related to national interests in defense or space exploration.[19]

1.2.5 *Mustard Gas Experiments*

In secret chemical weapons experiments conducted during World War II, the U.S. military experimented with a whopping 60,000 lowly ranked American troops in chambers filled with mustard gas. Subjects were oblivious of the consequence but were threatened with dishonorable discharge and military prison terms if they resisted. The tests evaluated protective equipment like gas masks and suits. They also compared the relative sensitivity of soldiers, including tests designed to look for racial differences. When those experiments were formally declassified in the 1990s, most of the affected human guinea pigs had passed on. More heinously, military records about the experimental subjects were intentionally muddied and incomplete with no identifying information, such as Social Security Numbers and addresses (to encumber later investigation). Consequently, the few surviving subjects who are today in their 80s and 90s – though still suffering from impacts of those chemical tests – (or their relatives), cannot be easily identified for appropriate compensation, due to burden of proof.[20]

---

19 Ibid, p. 44. Also, refer to the "Roadmap to the Project," DOE *Openness: Human Radiation Experiment*. Viewed on May 14, 2014 at http://www.rst2.edu/ties/radon/ramfordu/pdffiles/med8.pdf.

20 Read (and hear) more reports by Caitlin Dickerson, WWII Secret Mustard Gas Testing, *NPR*, at http://www.npr.org/2015/06/22/415194765/u-s-troops-tested-by-race-in-secret-world-war-ii-chemical-experiments, and http://www.npr.org/2015/06/23/416408655/the-vas-broken-promise-to-thousands-of-vets-exposed-to-mustard-gas. Accessed on July 16, 2015.

1.2.6 *Thalidomide*

Either partly because of its worldwide disastrous impact, or partly because of circumstances surrounding its original purpose (or both), the secrecy shrouding the real reason for the development of this pill may yet to be definitively made clear. The German pharmaceutical company Grünenthal is said to have developed it in Germany in 1944 as an antidote to nerve gases such as sarin; prior to which it was first synthesized by British scientists at the University of Nottingham in 1949.[21] But it was introduced into the market in Germany in 1957 as a wonder drug for insomnia, morning sickness (in pregnant women), coughs, colds and headaches.

By 1960 it had spread to the rest of the world, but was soon linked to miscarriages, severe deformities in children of mothers who took it in their first trimester of pregnancy. By this time more than 10,000 children in 46 countries had already been born with these defects. Though it had not been approved by the Food and Drug Administration, FDA, in the U.S., nevertheless, some doctors administered it to a selection of pregnant mothers (without their consent) on 'investigational basis.' Thus, 17 U.S. children were born with the defective conditions as a result.[22]

1.2.7 *Henry Beecher Report*

In 1966, Dr. Henry Beecher's article revealed the findings of his 10-year long study which jolted the medical community and repulsed the general public about the "thoughtless" and "careless" wide-spread ethical violations of the patients' rights in biomedical studies. With 22 examples to show (trimmed down from a much higher number) Beecher made evident that American investigators had "risked the health or the life of their subjects"[23] whose ages ranged from a few hours (from birth) to over 70 years – many of whom healthy, others in a variety of ill-health conditions. While citing inordinate drive for scientific progress and name recognition as motives for such experiments, Beecher also recalls Pope Pius XII admonitions that science should never be viewed as the highest value to which all other orders of value should be subordinated.[24]

21 For more navigate to *News Medical*, "History of Thalidomide" http://www.news-medical.net/health/History-of-Thalidomide.aspx. Viewed on May, 13, 2014.

22 Carl Coleman et al., p. 35.

23 Beecher, Henry. 1966. "Ethics and Clinical Research." *New England Journal of Medicine*, 274, 24:1356.

24 Ibid, p. 1354.

1.2.8 *Jewish Chronic Disease Hospital and Willowbrook Tests*

These two studies, though not identified but certainly part of Beecher's revelations, deserve a special mention due to their significance. In 1963, a study that received funding from the National Institutes of Health, NIH, was carried out by an unnamed Sloan-Kettering Cancer Research physician and conducted at the Jewish Chronic Disease Hospital during which live cancer cells were injected into 22 indigent, chronically ill, and debilitated elderly patients. "The participants were not informed that live cancer cells were being used or that the experiment was designed to measure the patient's ability to reject foreign cells – a test unrelated to their normal therapeutic program."[25]

Similarly, Willowbrook State School in New York was, between 1956 and 1971, the site of a Dr. Saul Krugman-led study which sought to "better understand the natural history of hepatitis and the effects of gamma globulin in preventing or moderating its effects."[26] The study subjects, all children, were deliberately infected with the hepatitis virus without their knowledge or assent (claims of signed consent forms by parents were unproven). In the end, even as this experiment established clear distinctions between Hepatitis A and B, a point for biomedical advancement,[27] however, its horrendous method did not go without condemnation.

Now, so much for instances of experimental callousness with human subjects. Obviously, the above cursory outline of the historical antecedents of experimentation with human subjects in the U.S. and elsewhere clearly projects a grim picture. While these few examples pertain only to biomedical testing, numerous other studies in fields such as the social sciences abound as well. It is beyond the ambits of this analysis to discuss them all. But with the lessons from these experiences gnawing at mankind's conscience, it was inevitable that some ethical codes of conduct would have to be formulated, if not to eliminate completely, to at least curtail future recurrence of similar abuses. As with most analyses with historical antecedents regarding Western medical ethics, Hippocrates/the Hippocratics often lead the way; in this case with the Oath (now better called the Hippocratic Pledge).[28] Below is a cursory mentioning of a few of the widely known provisions (in no particular order).

---

25 Carl Coleman et al., p. 39.

26 Ibid, p. 39.

27 Ibid, p. 39.

28 The World Medical Association. Accessed on October 12, 2017 from, https://www.wma.net/news-post/modern-physicians-pledge-approved-by-world-medical-association/.

1.3 Emergence of Research Ethics Codes

By default, most clinical trials, say of experimental drugs, start out with lab animals. But with greater level of confidence a series of phased[29] trials is introduced which involve human subjects but not without adherence to research ethics procedures. Underlying this fact is the degree of importance of the human person and the onus of responsibility we owe to human dignity.

The Nuremberg Military Tribunals under Control Council Law No. 10, 8–17, entailed a 140-day long proceeding, including the submission of about 1, 500 documents, testimonies of 85 witnesses, verdicts, and sentencing by presiding U.S. judges. Significantly, it also produced a terse landmark one-and-a half page framework – The Nuremberg Code – which aimed to guard against future human subject protection violations. It was the first of its kind and reads in part, "The voluntary consent of the human subject is absolutely essential. The duty and responsibility for ascertaining the quality of the consent rests upon each individual who initiates, directs or engages in the experiment. It is a duty and responsibility which may not be delegated to another with impunity."[30]

Next, the role of doctors in matters that determine rational actions in biomedical research is evident in the fashioning of mechanisms which ensure that similar issues are properly managed. Such is the case that was made by the World Medical Association in its *Declaration of Helsinki: Recommendations*

---

29 As defined by the U.S. National Institutes of Health, clinical trials (of drugs, medical devices, etc.) are conducted in a series of steps, called phases (four in all); each phase is designed to answer a separate research question. In phase I, for instance, researchers test a new drug or treatment in a small group of people for the first time to evaluate its safety, determine a safe dosage range, and identify side effects. As it progresses exponentially, in phase IV, studies are done after the drug or treatment has been marketed to gather information on the drug's effect in various populations and any side effects associated with long-term use. Get more details, "FAQ: ClinicalTrials.gov – Clinical Trial Phases," *NIH: US National Library of Science*, at http://www.nlm.nih.gov/services/ctphases.html. Viewed on October 28, 2013.

30 Trials of War Crime before the Nuremberg Military Tribunals under Control Council. 1949. No. 10, Vol. 2, pp. 181–182. Washington DC: U.S. Government Printing Office. Read more at Coleman et al. p. 16; and, "Special Focus," *U.S. Holocaust Memorial Museum*, at, http://www.ushmm.org/information/exhibitions/online-features/special-focus/doctors-trial. Viewed on May 14, 2014. It suffices to add here that though the Nuremberg Code was conceived and drafted by legal luminaries and even given the deceptive tag of a "Code," it doesn't actually have any legal bight. This flaw remains to be one of its main short comings and one wonders why such a milestone event could not produce a legally binding document.

Guiding Medical Doctors in Biomedical Research Involving Human Subjects, first adopted by the 18th World Medical Assembly in Helsinki, Finland, in 1964. This document has been revised multiple times since then to accommodate updates and shortcomings of previous ones.[31] The 37-point four-page document retains its usual elements which essentially stress the importance of ethical principles for medical research involving human subjects.

Also, the Good Clinical Practice, GCP, protocol that guides ethical research conducts originating in Europe is worthy of mention here. It is an international ethical and scientific quality standard for designing, conducting, recording and reporting trials that involve the participation of human subjects. Compliance with this standard provides public assurance that the rights, safety and well-being of trial subjects are protected, in keeping with the principles that have their origin in the Declaration of Helsinki and the World Medical Association (WMA).[32] In recognition that clinical development of medicines has become a global undertaking, the London-based European Medicines Agency, nurtured an initiative to collaborate with the USFDA. This procedure was launched in July 2009 and aimed to ensure "the protection of clinical-trial subjects in the context of the increasing globalization of clinical research."[33]

On the U.S. front, it is scarcely surprising given the history of research with human subjects, that regulations are plentiful. In comparing the culture of research ethics in Australia, Europe, and North America, Paul M. McNeill, an Australian attorney and ethicist, attests that the American research ethics climate is far more widely publicized, witnesses much more regulations, and that those regulations are more detailed than in any other country.[34] For a comprehensive understanding of this, an extended list of examples in support of McNeil's observation is appropriate:

- As noted in the Thalidomide saga, the impact cut across many countries. In the U.S., it "led to the passage, in late 1962, of the Kefauver-Harris

31 "Special Communication," *The Journal of American Medical Association.* Published online October 19, 2013. Also see, https://www.wma.net/policies-post/wma-declaration-of-helsinki-ethical-principles-for-medical-research-involving-human-subjects/.

32 Refer to the "Good Clinical Practice Compliance," *European Medicines Agency,* at, http://www.ema.europa.eu/ema/index.jsp?curl=pages/regulation/general/general_content_000072.jsp. Viewed on May 21, 2014.

33 Ibid.

34 McNeil, Paul. 1989. "Research Ethics Review in Australia, Europe, and North America IRB: Ethics and Human Research," *The Hastings Center*, 11, 3:4.

Amendments to the earlier federal Food, Drug and Cosmetic Act of 1938, strengthening the FDA's control of drug experimentation on humans."[35]

- The National Institutes of Health's Policies for the Protection of Human Subjects, which were first issued in 1966, attained regulatory status and were promulgated on May 30, 1974 by the Department of Health, Education and Welfare (DHEW). They established the Institutional Review Board (IRB) which are empowered to approve research protocols that guaranteed adequate protection for human subjects in research.[36]
- In July 1974, the National Research Act created the National Commission for the Protection of Human Subjects of Biomedical and Behavioral Research. The Commission "issued reports and recommendations identifying the basic ethical principles that should underlie the conduct of biomedical and behavioral research involving human subjects and recommending guidelines to ensure that research is conducted in accordance with those principles."[37] The Commission's report was a precursor to The Belmont Report.
- Research ethics and bioethics as a whole are indebted to The Belmont Report for originally formulating three basic ethical principles (a.k.a., principlism) that have become a *condicio sine qua non* in any conduct of research involving human subjects. As a moral decision-making approach, principlism is now however more often associated with Tom Beauchamp and James Childress – two most prominent stalwarts of bioethics. But having borrowed the idea from The Belmont Report,[38] the two ethicists extended the theory to four pillars of *respect for autonomy* (a norm of respecting the decision-making capacities of autonomous persons); *non-maleficence* (a norm of avoiding the causation of harm); *beneficence* (a group of norms for providing benefits and balancing benefits against risks and costs); and, *justice* (a group of norms for distributing benefits, risks, and costs fairly).[39]

---

35 Coleman et al, pp. 35–36. Also see, Bren, L. 2001. *Frances Oldham Kelsey: FDA Medical Reviewer Leaves Her Mark on History*, "Consumer Updates," *FDA* at http://www.fda.gov/fdac/features/2001/201_kelsey.html.

36 "The History of the Human Subject Protection System." Read more at the McLaren Health Care at http://www.mclaren.org/northernmichigan/TheHistoryoftheHumanSubjectsProtectionSystemirb.aspx. Viewed on May 9, 2014.

37 Ibid.

38 The name is abridged from the following, The Belmont Report: Ethical Principles and Guidelines for the Protection of Human Subjects of Research. It was so named after the Belmont Conference Center at the Smithsonian Institution where the discussions which resulted in its formulation were held.

39 Beauchamp, Tom and Childress, James, 2012, p. 38.

- Further still, following the recommendations of the National Commission's report in 1981, both the Department of Health and Human Services (DHHS, formerly DHEW) and the FDA promulgated significant revisions of their human subjects' regulations. "The DHHS regulations are codified at Title 45 Part 46 of the Code of Federal Regulations. Those 'basic' regulations became final on January 16, 1981, and were revised effective March 4, 1983, and June 18, 1991. The June 18, 1991, revision involved the adoption of the Federal Policy for the Protection of Human Subjects. The Federal Policy [a.k.a. Common Rule] was promulgated by the 16 federal agencies that conduct, support, or otherwise regulate human subjects research; the FDA also adopted [some parts of] its provisions. As implied by its title, the Federal Policy is designed to make uniform the human subjects' protection system (Common Rule) in all relevant federal agencies and departments."[40] The DHHS Office of Human Research Protections has further modified this rule for 2018 onwards.
- By an Executive Order 12975, the U.S. president established the National Bioethics Advisory Commission on October 3, 1995.[41] The NBAC's charter expired on October 3, 2001, nevertheless it provided advice and made recommendations to the National Science and Technology Council and to other appropriate government entities on a range of matters; among them was the appropriate ethical conduct in research involving human participants. Not surprisingly, this was mandated by President Clinton, who as I noted earlier, tendered a heartfelt apology for the Tuskegee atrocity.
- To speak specifically on the powers of FDA in the protection of human research subjects, Stuart Nightingale, FDA associate commissioner for health affairs, indicates that it is "an outgrowth and expression of FDA's unique responsibilities vis-a-vis research in general and clinical research in particular."[42] Thus, in its regulatory mission, the FDA reviews applications for market products which have a direct, often vital effect on human health and welfare. Drugs and biologics, medical devices, radiation-emitting equipment, and food and color additives, are examples of such products. To approve them, FDA is required to closely examine the procedure and

40 McLaren Health Care's "The History of the Human Subject Protection System." Read more at the http://www.mclaren.org/northernmichigan/TheHistoryoftheHumanSubjectsProtectionSystemirb.aspx. Viewed on May 9, 2014.

41 National Bioethics Advisory Commission. 2001. "Ethical and Policy Issues in Research Involving Human Participants."

42 Nightingale, Stuart. 1983. "The Food and Drug Administration's Role in the Protection of Human Subjects." *IRB: Ethics and Human Research*, 5, 1:6.

results of research conducted and paid for by interested parties outside the government.[43]

Apart from the historical events dotting America's not-so-rosy record with biomedical human experimentation, there are also political and cultural factors, including individuality and individual rights dispositions which join up to shape the field. Bioethics itself is an intellectual and cultural phenomenon, which rose from the ashes of aforementioned medical scandals that seemed to culminate in the 1970s. It was a turning point decade marked by other landmark movements such as the anti-Viet Nam war and the environmental movements both of which are rooted in the civil rights movement.[44]

In addition to the factors already named, the following has to be underscored: the scope of governmental influence over the regulatory process of ethics review. This is unique like no other. For instance, the U.S. federal government has for long devised a mechanism for channeling research monies directly by designated departments. This has meant that the government exercises greater oversight over disbursed funds for intended research purposes.[45]

All of this lend credence to the claim that the U.S. arena is head and shoulders above all other countries in just about all considerations in biomedical research, including, those that involve human subjects. However, it remains to be seen how far that goes. For instance, despite the well-established regulations and guidelines, water-tight responsibility for human subjects in research are still elusive. In fact, by some uncanny twist one might deduce that the legal, social, cultural and political structures that are in place, and crowned by burning economic reasons, might account for the accelerated rate of outsourcing of biomedical studies to other places like the Global South. In the section that follows, I discuss some of the convoluted implications that have become the by-products of off-shoring and outsourcing of biomedical research.

43 Ibid, p. 6.

44 Other captivating details of the historical metamorphosis of the bioethics field, starting with the invention of the word "bioethics," can be found in "The History of Bioethics: An Essay Review" by Martensen, R., *Journal of the History of Medicine*, 56: 168–175, 2001; "The Origins and Evolution of Bioethics: Some Personal Reflections" by Pellegrino, E., *Kennedy Institute of Ethics Journal*, 9.1: 73–88, 1999; and Judy Andre's *Bioethics as Practice*, The University of North Carolina Press, 2002.

45 McNeil, p. 4. More of this history has been traced by Jercker, Jonsen, and Pearlman, (1997), *Bioethics: An Introduction*; and, Jonsen, Albert, (1998) *The Birth of Bioethics*.

1.4 Outsourcing of Clinical Trials

The release of the report, "The globalization of clinical trials: A growing challenge in protecting human subjects" in September 2001 by the Inspector General of the U.S. Department of Health and Human Services, set a historic milestone in biomedical research.[46] Right off the bat, this report succumbed to admitting at least two major issues. One, the decades-long inadequacy of oversight systems that existed for human subject protections particularly, given the emergent globalizing trend that I have noted. Two, and drawing on a similar report the department did the previous year, it is an admission that industry-sponsored research has taken the lead in swiftly moving clinical trials mostly from the Global North to the Global South (of which Africa forms a significant swath). Many of the government-sponsored ones also have either willingly followed in tow or been dragged along, albeit, kicking and screaming.

Other findings from the DHHS inquiry are that while sponsors have expanded research sites into many countries that appear to have limited experience in clinical trials, FDA cannot assure the same level of human subject protections in foreign trials as domestic ones. It therefore recommended a barrage of measures. For instance, that FDA should obtain more information about the performance of foreign institutional review boards by working with the regulatory authorities in foreign countries; help foreign boards build capacity; encourage sponsors to obtain attestations from foreign investigators; encourage greater sponsor monitoring by encouraging more rigorous monitoring of foreign research sites by sponsors and their agents; and, develop a database to track the growth and location of foreign research. In addition, they urge the Office for Human Research Protections to exert leadership and encourage participation of IRBs in a voluntary accreditation system.[47]

These recommendations are inherently inadequate simply because they are, *recommendations*, not directives backed by enforceable legal sanction. Statutory provisions establishing the DHHS apparently do not allow for enforcement of such provisions. Also, this set of recommendations falls flat on its face mainly because much of the foreign-based research are industry-sponsored; so even if Office for Human Research Protections were to exert sanctions, they are limited mostly to government-sponsored research which are currently in the

46 U.S. Department of Health and Human Services, Office of Inspector General, Janet Rehnquist, Inspector General report; "The Globalization of Clinical Trials a Growing Challenge in Protecting Human Subjects." September, 2001.

47 Ibid, p. iii.

minority. The hamstrings that these recommendations suffer could be compared to those of international standards, which are essentially principle-based, voluntary, not embedded in enforceable legal instruments, and lack aggressive quality to verify implementation process. Not surprisingly, these are consequences that naturally flow from such bureaucratic caveats.

It seems appropriate at this stage to pause and take a bite of the question posed earlier: Who is responsible for human subjects [when experiments travel]? To risk a hackneyed answer, common sense dictates that all clinical research must be primed to abide by any and all approved ethical codes (international and local) to protect human subjects. The primary responsibilities of clinical investigators are to protect the rights, integrity and confidentiality of trial subjects (*everywhere* and at all times). And for researchers with U.S. federal government and industry funding, the international good clinical practice guidelines, etc., must in addition be complied with. But that's not all.

To apprise the reader with what is at stake, let me offer instead a flip side to that question: Why are research subjects' protection in international research so important now? Richard Carpentier, of the Canadian National Council on Ethics in Human Research and FOCUS Secretariat raised a similarly instructive poser and followed with equally instructive answers that we are keen to anticipate. Protections are increasingly important because of a host of reasons: research activities are increasing more than ever before; multiple ethical breaches are happening more frequently; research is moving into countries with less experience and infrastructures; research is less and less in control of academic/public institutions and more in control of for-profit corporations; and lastly, there is a crying need to create and sustain trust.[48]

Current research ethics guidelines are universal, at least they are crafted to largely apply universally. But, later I will argue that the assumptions implicit in the mainstream (Western) ethical framework that make claim to universal validity are not shared by many non-Western cultures. For instance, the mainstream research ethics purports to adhere to the principlist quartet (autonomy, beneficence, non-maleficence and justice) which are inherently linked to Western individualistic notions of personhood, whereas the rest of the world, particularly Africa, sees the person not as an isolated individual, but as a part of the community which is embedded in kinship, group and community. So, by "universal application" I imply that human subjects in research anywhere deserve basic protection across the board without discrimination.

48 Richard Carpentier made this point in a keynote joint public presentation in 2001 along with Janet Rehnquist, Inspector General, USDHHS, and Daniel Lenvinson, Inspector General, Office of Inspector General.

Since the Nuremburg Code, the Belmont Report, Declaration of Helsinki, DoH, (or The Council for International Organizations of Medical Sciences, CIOMS), etc., the primary aim has always been to guarantee the protection of human subjects. I will reserve for another time a proper assessment of how far that protection has been attained.

By implication, I am presupposing or have gone beyond asking, why are clinical trials off-shoring? If I must reiterate, the phenomenon of off-shoring comes mainly at the instance of globalization – a fleeting concept that assumes different meanings depending on the context. For instance, it can mean "a laudable development uniting humankind or an epidemic crushing the vulnerable peoples of the earth."[49] As I have mentioned earlier, it also connotes a phenomenon that enables entities to escape sanctions in certain locales and exploit loopholes in other places for maximization of quick profits.

A contemporary African philosopher, Theophilus Okere, thinks that the intended positives that might have emerged from globalization have by some unfortunate way assumed a one-way traffic whereby the world is being unified essentially by westernizing or assimilating western values (individualism and materialism as ideal). It seems also to have become a process of unifying socio-economic systems (democracy and capitalism) as a way of defining success and progress. Okere further reasons that it is a type of war by another means; a subtle war, obviously raging but rather surreptitiously and aims to eviscerate the identity of other cultures, and threatens to reduce the world to a drab monotony.[50]

But, despite the apparent sidetracking, globalization, rightly applied should actually signal the realization of both the diversity (ecological, biological, cultural, and linguistic) and the interdependence of the various parts of the world. Godfrey Tangwa elucidates nicely that globalization arises as well from the simple realization that the "dangers facing the world as a whole, even if emanating largely from only a small part of it, can best be tackled only from a global perspective."[51]

All of this conveys a sense of legitimate activities operating across national boundaries. And whether or not you know it, like it, or understand it,

---

49 Sladikas, Milto and Schroeder, Doris. 2005. "Too Early for Global Ethics?" *Cambridge Quarterly of Healthcare Ethics*, 14:404.

50 Okere, Theophilus. 2005. *Philosophy, Culture and Society in Africa*. Enugu: Victojo Productions, pp. 60–61.

51 Tangwa, Godfrey. 2004. "Some African Reflections on Biomedical and Environmental Ethics." *A Companion to African Philosophy. Wiredu,* Kwasi (Ed.). Massachusetts: Blackwell Publishing Ltd. p. 387.

globalization has since become unavoidable. Which leaves me with the trite conclusion that literally everything is already swept up by the globalization phenomenon. Yes, research ethics too.

Thus, the fact that transnational biomedical research has increased in scope (particularly from the Global North to the Global South), thanks mostly to throes of globalization, is a long established fact.[52,53] As a consequence, evidence of concern and substantial debate about the ethics of research in the developing countries where they are off-shored to has worried many analysts.[54,55] The application of principlism abroad (having evolved out of Western philosophical traditions) in research ethics and bioethics in general, in disregard of alternative and competing ethical frameworks, and different civilizational traditions and socio-political conditions, seems to present its own significant challenges as well.[56] A catalogue of other concerns about biomedical studies that are initiated in the industrialized world and conducted in the emerging world are widespread. They include, the appeal to harvest ignorant, willing, and desperate subjects for expeditious trial which leads to early registration of drugs and ultimately the enhancement of considerable corporate profits. But in all of this, Ruth Macklin[57] has posed the question that I have asked here as well: How does (or should) the research ethics standards apply and who does (or should) the experimenter answer to, the local or international regulatory authorities, or both? I would let the reader ruminate over those questions which I will answer momentarily with a detailed case study.

Hence, I want to introduce a real life public health scenario and relate it to my analysis of responsibility. With this test case, I claim that in public health,

52 Fitzgerald, D. Wasuna, Angela, and Pape, Jean. 2003. "Ten Questions Institutional Review Boards Should Ask When Reviewing International Clinical Research Protocols." IRB: Ethics and Human Research, *The Hastings Center.*

53 National Bioethics Advisory Commission Report: Ethical and Policy Issues in International Research. 2001. *The Hastings Center*, 23, 4: 9–12.

54 Emanuel, Ezekiel, et al. 2004. "What Makes Clinical Research in Developing Countries Ethical? The Benchmarks of Ethical Research." *The Journal of Infectious Diseases*, 189, 5: 930–937.

55 Fitzgerald, Daniel and Wasuna, Angela. 2005. "Away from Exploitation and Towards Engagement: An Ethical Compass for Medical." *The Journal of Law, Medicine & Ethics*, 33, 3: 559–565.

56 Brodwin, Paul. 2001. "Pluralism and Politics in Global Bioethics Education." *Annals of Behavioral Science and Medical Education.* 7, 2: 80–86. Also, Emanuel, Ezekiel, et al. (2004) similarly argue that "The Persistence of Controversies on Such Issues Reflects, in Part, the Fact That Existing Ethical Guidelines Can be Interpreted in Multiple Ways, are Sometimes Contradictory, or Rely on Unstated, Yet Controversial, Ethical Principles," p. 930.

57 Macklin, Ruth. 2004. *Double Standards in Medical Research in Developing Countries.* Cambridge, UK: Cambridge University Press.

just as in medical ethics generally, responsibility is both subliminal as well as overt. In the case of population-based research, the concern is that biomedical scientists, while riding on readily available trust, might sometimes be inclined to renege on their charge with responsibility and force unwanted procedures on the public. In doing so, patient-subjects are made to sacrifice personal dignity, autonomy, safety, liberty, and cultural identity in the name of doing research for the public benefit. This seems to be the case with the experimental drug, *Trovan*. As I will make clear shortly, the Pfizer experiment may be emblematic of all that should not happen particularly when clinical trials travel abroad. It includes hubris, disrespect for other cultures, apparent emphasis on profit, use of patient-subjects solely as means, disregard for local authority, and betrayal of trust; all of which are hallmarks of irresponsibility.

1.5 Trovan Test Case[58]

In 1996, concurrent epidemics of cerebro-spinal and bacterial meningitis, measles, and cholera were affecting children in Kano, a northern Nigerian city. This coincided with the trial phase in the development of Trovafloxacin (or Trovan), a quinolone antibiotic by Pfizer. The American pharmaceutical giant learned of this outbreak in the news and dispatched a research team to a local hospital providing treatment. Pfizer administered Trovan to a large number of pediatric patients as part of its effort to determine the effectiveness of the experimental drug in treating meningitis. The drug had never been tested on children. All the children in the study were picked from among the long lines of people seeking care. The experiment took place at the same hospital where a team of Mèdicins Sans Frontières was already providing free treatment with Ceftriaxone, a gold standard antibiotic medication internationally recommended for treating meningitis.

A Nigeria government's investigative report later blamed the drug trial for a combination of effects ranging from adverse drug reaction, adverse events, to serious adverse events.[59] For instance, in the immediate aftermath of the trial, 11 of those trial subjects died; many more suffer (ongoing) permanent disabilities such as brain damage, paralysis, muteness, slurred speech, and

58 This test case happened in the mid-1990's, before the afore-mentioned DHHS report. But, apparently, incidents like this might have informed that report.

59 For the definitions of these terms, see "Key to Abbreviations/Terms" in this book. Definitions were culled from the International Conference on Harmonization of Technical Requirements, for Registration of Pharmaceuticals for Human Use, ICH, Harmonized Tripartite Guideline for Good Clinical Practice E6(R1), Step 4 version, June 10, 1996.

blindness.[60] A series of law suits by the victims and the Nigerian government (filed in the U.S. under the Alien Tort Claims Act) commenced in 2001,[61] but was aborted by the U.S. Supreme Court in the fall of 2010. Pfizer had struck a $75-million out-of-court settlement for claims related to the experiment. In late 2010, Pfizer also offered to build a $25-million hospital in the city, a gesture aimed to further appease the people. Pfizer made the first compensation payment to Nigerian families affected. The amount, $175,000 (£108,000) each went to four families in the first of a series of payments it was expected to make.[62]

The wrinkle on this matter could be that the drug maker's move may have stymied or effectively squelched every chance to either validate or dismiss a laundry list of allegations which include that:

- Pfizer took advantage of the chaos from the medical crises as an opportunity to quickly conduct the study (a potentially dangerous treatment) on young children, something it had been unable to obtain permission to do elsewhere.
- Pfizer obtained no informed assent from any of the children participating in the trial (or consent from their parents).
- Pfizer provided no explanation to the children or their parents that the treatment was experimental and that they were free to refuse it in favor of the known effective treatment available at the same hospital free of charge.
- Pfizer never received the necessary approvals (either from the Nigerian government or the hospital administration) to conduct the research, but when the FDA began to conduct an audit of Pfizer's Trovan records, suddenly a forged letter dated March 1996 surfaced stating that the hospital's ethics committee had approved the Trovan study. (The investigation established that at the time the trial took place, the hospital neither had an ethics committee nor a letterhead on which the (Pfizer's) letter appeared).

Unanswered posers still linger as to possible motives: is it for reasons of advancing biomedical science; promoting corporate (and/or individual) record, achievement and glory; or enhancing corporate wealth? For one, Trovan was

60 In "Panel Faults Pfizer in '96 Clinical Trial in Nigeria – Unproven Drug Tested in Children" Joe Stevens of the *Washington Post* relates the controversial saga in the edition on Sunday May 7, 2006; p. A01.

61 *The New York Times*, August 30, 2001.

62 See more at, http://www.sunnewsonline.com/webpages/news/national/2010/dec/02/national-02-12-2010-005.htm. Accessed December 02, 2010. Also, see *BBC News*, http://www.bbc.co.uk/news/world-africa-14493277. Accessed April 11, 2013.

primed to be Pfizer's next major profit gusher, estimated to net billions of dollars in yearly sales if approved by the FDA. Meanwhile, victims of that experiment have continued to suffer (even as I write) and to die in their twenties; reigniting debates concerning ethics of biomedical research that involve patient-subjects. Some of the immediate impacts are the scar of suspicion and erosion of trust – two prime factors that are linked to the near failure of age-long vaccination campaigns in the adjoining regions of that country. As such this Moslem-dominated area has harbored and witnessed the recurrence of preventable diseases, such as polio, that have long been wiped out in most parts of the world.

Such is one instance where lack of faith in scientists might justify opposition to the technologies their work has spawned. Public trust – an indispensable ingredient in the success of any clinical trials – can be eroded as a result of some or all of these reasons: if there is persistent perception that subjects of clinical trials are there as a means to an end; if there is the perception or even suspicion that only lip service is paid to ethics; if clinicians are not upfront as to the nature, the risks, possible benefits of the research; and, if or where conflicts of interests might lie. Concerns could rise even further when these facts are placed on the back of a research finding from a survey of more than 200 developing countries which concluded that one-quarter of clinical trials carried out in the Global South do not undergo any kind of ethical review in the host nations.[63]

In spite of the lessons of history – recall the many push factors that forced the formulation of research ethics guidelines and codes, etc., and the vow of 'never again under our watch' – when a clinical trial disaster recurs, as in the Pfizer-Nigeria example, we are bound to return to the soul-searching question of: how did we get it wrong, *again*? The broader philosophical prodding could be the reason why philosophers have urged that epistemologists must make use of results from the sciences that study human reasoning in pursuing epistemological questions. In other words, epistemology should become a branch of psychology and charged with not worrying whether what we claim to be the facts are true; epistemologists should rather be concerned with figuring out what the mechanisms are by which we believe by taking up the empirical psychological study of our cognitive processes.

In the case of human-subjects, we ought to place in tandem the epistemic content of biomedical training and its application in the field of clinical practice in order to evaluate their value and relevance in terms of pursuing

63 Dawson, L. et al. 2004. "Ethical Review of Health Research: A Perspective from Developing Country Researchers." *Journal of Medical Ethics*, 30, 1:68.

and attaining mutual goals. Unfortunately, while this is supposed to result in a meeting point, a bifurcation emerges instead: there is a difference between treating others respectfully (for instance, paying back trust) because one recognizes the need for their active engagement in and with one's work, and treating them respectfully because to do otherwise (irresponsible behavior) would be either morally wrong or instrumentally troublesome, or both. It may be fair to say that clinicians in the Pfizer-Nigeria test case apparently squandered the faith entrusted in them by failing to demonstrate epistemic interest in their subjects.

To act with epistemic interest assumes the intrinsic value of persons; it doesn't seem like that was displayed here. Acting with epistemic interest, nay repaying trust, is one way to earn public trust (I will return to this subject later). Meanwhile, I wish to briefly argue that the clinician's training must in no way isolate him/her from his/her object (or in this case, subject) of knowledge. The opposite is rather urged. The proof of the efficacy of the scientific product which is the result of endless lab hours and of mental labor, must be guided to make a reasoned landing in the field of practice. That, to use the common parlance, is where the rubber meets the road.

> Because knowledge is meant to apply to, and to be applicable in the world outside the laboratory, it is important to ask what the knowledge is knowledge *of*. Real problems arise about the applicability of research findings beyond the research setting, and one way of framing those problems is in terms of whether, and to what extent, the objects of the research are relevantly different from the objects in the wider world they are taken to exemplify.[64]

As a related matter, I observe with glee that the trust analysis Annette Baier[65] eloquently proposed in her celebrated essay "Trust, and anti-trust" makes references to (among other things) not just individual human beings or groups of people, but denotes also the perspective that recognizes 'legal persons' natural or artificial, such as firms (i.e., business enterprises) and nations. It is hard to ignore the 'person' of Pfizer and the share force of its enormous influence in the international community. Given this, or even in spite of it, it is intriguing that Pfizer (whose clout on the world stage easily surpasses that of many individual countries) would as it seems, apply tricky, deceptive, and hoodwinking tactics to recruit pediatric patient-subjects for the experimental drug. Adding

64 Scheman, N. 2009. "Narrative, Complexity, and Context: Anatomy as an Epistemic Value." *Naturalized Bioethics*, Cambridge: Cambridge University Press, p. 111.

65 Baier, Annette. 1986. "Trust and Antitrust." *Ethics*, 96, 2: 231–260.

to that, it seems inappropriate that Pfizer finds it suitable to do in an African country something it couldn't do anywhere in the Global North.

Added to the medical privilege are matters of racial contractarianism and vestiges of colonial mentality and neo-coloniality. Since a forceful tactic for maintaining cognitive authority and control is to insist on the conceit that one's knowledge trumps that of the other, some clinical investigators from the Global North often confirm the perception that they either don't understand the local community they have come to work in or simply don't care to trust them; widening further the chasm between them and their patient-subjects who they should primarily care for. In consonant with Eva Kittay's[66] discussion of arrogant imposition of one's own values on others, this could be seen as acting out of hubris. It is an epistemic tunnel vision that detracts from the goals of ethics of care. Even as the interests of the patient-subject may sometimes yield to the interests of science, in the trenchant words of Jay Katz, "this revolutionary development has not been accompanied by a thoroughgoing re-examination of physicians' ethical obligations in a post-Hippocratic age."[67]

1.6 Concluding Thoughts

To address the question that this chapter poses, "Who is Responsible for Human Subjects When Experiments Travel?" I purposely revisited the history of experimentation with humans for some background. The not-so-colorful picture led to, at various times and on a variety of platforms nationally and internationally, the composition of numerous regulations, polices, assurances and guidelines which aim to protect human subjects in research. To reiterate, prior to the now familiar regulations and guidelines to protect human subjects in research, there were documented abuses. As I have made apparent, the glaring historical antecedents in experimentation with human subjects prompted the formulation of research ethics principles to guide every study at every stage, *everywhere*.

Nonetheless, it is my contention that with certain developments such as globalization, the nature and terrain of our actions in biomedical research

66 Kittay, Eva. 2009. "Ideal Theory Bioethics and the Exclusion of People with Severe Cognitive Disabilities." *Naturalized Bioethics: Toward Responsible Knowing and Practice,* (eds.) Hilde Lindemann, Marian Verkerk and Margaret Walker. Cambridge University Press, p. 235.

67 Katz, Jay. 2005. "Informed Consent to Research: Human Experimentation and Human Rights" *The Ethics and Regulation of Research with Human Subjects*, (eds.) Coleman, C. et al., New Jersey: Mathew Bender and Company, p. 308.

have changed. As a consequence, it's only logical that this change warrants a corresponding change that fundamentally touches on the conduct, ethics, and cultural shift in carrying out biomedical research. My trend of thought here seems to fit succinctly with Hans Jonas' characterization of the ethics of an endangered future when he says:

> This [is] not merely in the sense that new objects of action have added to the case material on which received rules of conduct are to be applied, but in the more radical sense that qualitatively novel nature of certain of our actions has opened up a whole new dimension of ethical as well as relevance for which there is no precedent in the standards and cannons of traditional ethics.[68]

I have also noted the mismatch in adherence to rule compliance between on one hand, the industrialized world (Global North) which is adequately structured for sufficient monitoring, and on the other hand, the industrializing world (Global South) which is hamstrung by inadequate or non-existent infrastructure to aid monitoring and compliance. As a corollary, the effective compliance regimen in the Global North, coupled with the excuse of globalization have meant that increasing amounts of research efforts are conducted in the Global South having been conceived in the Global North. And with this development come untold consequences in the recipient countries.

As far as the history of biomedical research goes, the importance given to human value and the protection of that value, are never in question. I have argued that the intension for which the now familiar series of guidelines and codes for human subject protection ought to keep pace with the emerging socio-economic world trends, for instance, globalization. Thus, there must not be application of double standards irrespective of the study site. In fact, rather than do less, research teams should expect to lean over backwards and to do much more when experiments are off-shored by incorporating both international and local guidelines and codes (as much as possible). But with the Nigeria-Pfizer example, one wonders why some foreign-sponsored biomedical research tend to apply a different set of rules, particularly, in regard to protection of human subjects, that they would otherwise not do in stricter climes.

Authors have noted the opportunity for exploitation[69] of the weak and the poor by the powerful and the rich as attempts to address health research

68 Jonas, Hans. 1981. "Technology and Responsibility: The Ethics of an Endangered Future" in *Responsibilities to Future Generations*, New York: Prometheus Books, p. 23.

69 Read more by Hyder, A. et al. 2004. "Ethical Review of Health Research: A Perspective from Developing Country Researchers" *Journal of Medical Ethics*, 30:68–72.

issues increasingly hinge on the intertwining of the needs of different countries at the international level. What had been hoped to possibly pose a challenge in the distant future has all but suddenly enveloped us as national borders and boundaries are made ever more porous and transgressed by technologies and trade.

A truth-apt attempt would be to starkly restate that the guidelines are just what they are, *guidelines*. Extra efforts would have to be made, as Fitzgerald et al., suggest (something that hints on inculcation of virtue ethics), for any meaningful outcome to be realized in this area. For instance, they prescribe a 10-point list of questions IRBs must seek satisfactory answers for before international clinical research protocols are approved.

The questions include: Does the research protocol address the ethical challenges of conducting research in a developing country? Is the purpose of the research responding to the health needs of the host country? Does anyone else in the host country know about the research? Are the risks to volunteers acceptable in the social context of the host country?[70]

Arguing along the same line, Ezekiel Emanuel, et al., expand on such issues as unwavering respect for recruited participants and study communities before, during and long after studies have been conducted. They underscore enduring obligations researchers should have to participants, former participants, and the host community.[71] The challenge of striking a balance between the need to protect the subjects, and to reduce the much-resented bureaucratic burden on field officers remains a big one. In spite of frequent complaints and accusations by researchers against independent gatekeepers or IRBs for bogging down their studies through 'micromanaging consent forms' and research protocols, and 'fretting unnecessarily' about psychological harm that might be caused by asking people questions, whether in the lab or in the field; I'm inclined to stick with the recommendation to be steadfast and focused on the importance of oversight so as to get things right. I agree with Emanuel and colleagues in fending off any possible insinuation or objection to the suggested

70 Fitzgerald, Daniel et al. 2003. pp. 14–18. Also, see Fitzgerald, Daniel and Wasunna, Angela. 2005. "Away from Exploitation and Towards Engagement: An Ethical Compass for Medical Researchers Working in Resource-Poor Countries." *The Journal of Law, Medicine & Ethics;* 33, 3:559ff. Also see, "Ethical Oversight of Research in Developing Countries" by Kass, Nancy et al. 2003. Ethics and Human Research, *The Hastings Center* 25, 2: 1–10.

71 Emanuel, Ezekiel, Wendler, David, Killen, Jack, Grady, Christine. 2004. "What Makes Clinical Research in Developing Countries Ethical? The Benchmarks of Ethical Research." *The Journal of Infectious Diseases*, 189, 5: 930–937. Chicago: The University of Chicago Press. For more on fair benefits, refer to El Setouhy, Maged et al. 2004. "Moral Standards for Research in Developing Countries from 'Reasonable Availability' to 'Fair Benefits'" *The Hastings Center Report*, 34, 3: 17–27.

framework as another layer of barriers to research in developing countries. Emmanuel et al's benchmark clearly provides explicit and systematic delineation of steps for conscientious researchers doing work in the Global South so as to make coherent the already widely accepted principles and benchmarks in the Nuremberg Code, the DoH, the Belmont Report, etc.[72]

No doubt, the answer to the question for this chapter has been made apparent from the foregoing. Put differently, I have proved my thesis (even as it is axiomatic) that researchers must abide by research ethics doctrines and are deemed fully responsible for all human subjects in their study whether or not experiments travel (outsourced/off-shored) or are conducted locally. In many circumstances, stakes might even be higher along with level of responsibility when research scientists engage with local authorities (at clinical trial sites) and should take on additional rules. Besides, if the historical significance of Hippocrates is anything, the following attribution to him should find resonance in contemporary biomedical research arena: it is more important to know that a person has a disease than to ask who it is that has the disease. In other words, it is irrelevant who it is that has disease, what is relevant in an unbiased healthcare delivery process is finding ways to treat or cure the person with disease.

Thus far, I have demonstrated that as the research arenas in the Global North continue to double down with regulation, a reality that has been nudged further afield by the phenomenon of globalization, researchers tend to cast their net farther off-shore in search of soft targets, including Africa, which is notorious for lax or non-existent apparati for such experiments. And operating in structurally weak environments for proper enforcement of research ethics guidelines, some researchers tend to feel no urgent obligation to strictly abide by widely established ethical guidelines and principles, and to renege on the charge to be adequately responsible to human research subjects.

But for the grander picture for the future, I have alluded that research ethics, as reflected in the mainstream principles, is not a one-size-fits-all template that you can simply conjure up and apply at will. We are at a point, indeed, that the cry grows loudest for a new deal. Like John Passmore who argued for a new morality to deal with the future of our environment, I argue here for a new perspective which can only grow out of emerging mindset, just because, unlike a speculative hypothesis, it is pointless unless it actually shapes our conduct and the way forward. But, on the evidence of it, it might not be completely shocking to see that our attitudes might already be primed for one choice: change. In the main, "that the 'new morality' would be a natural outcome of a change that is already in process, which can now be hastened by exhortation

72 Ibid, p. 936.

or argument."[73] A pointer to this promise of a new direction can be gleaned from the WHO-sponsored study, *Guidance Framework for Testing of Genetically Modified Mosquitoes*, the relevant parts of which I have reviewed in Chapter 2. The WHO compendium outlays a set of genuine clinical trial process that clearly goes beyond the individualistic basis of principlism and recognizes the crucial role of other cultures in the understanding of personhood as a concept that is embedded in the community.

It is a considerable presumption that given the current trend, the task of meeting the challenges of human subject protections in today's globalized biomedical research environment requires a concerted and well-coordinated international commitment. Because all ethics is local, one is spared from getting giddy in an attempt to figure out appropriate ways to integrate ethical systems of the nearly 200-member states of the WHO countries (and regions) along with their multiple political, social, cultural, and economic vagaries. It has thus been noted that following the U.S. Inspector General's continued exhortation, the new thinking is likely to come into fruition if we are prepared to be more tenacious in constantly reminding ourselves of some basic facts:

- International guidelines and national law[s] alone will not suffice. Without a systematic approach to information gathering and capacity building, standards alone will not achieve greater protections for research subjects through independent and competent ethical review *in all countries* (my emphasis).
- Given the enormous complexity of cultural variations, national laws, and local medical and research practices, local knowledge and local engagement are essential to develop ethical review. In addition, the principles of bioethics and the need for sustained development demand that responsibility be born at the local level, as close to the patient as possible.[74]

I concur.

73 Passmore, John. 1974. *Man's Responsibility for Nature: Ecological Problems and Western Traditions*. New York: Charles Scribner's Sons, p. 111.

74 Crawley, Francis, Esber, Elaine, Lin, Melody, Karbwan, Juntra. 2002. "Ethical Review and the Globalization of Clinical Trials." *Applied Clinical Trials Online*. Viewed on June 18, 2014 at http://www.appliedclinicaltrialsonline.com/appliedclinicaltrials/EU/Ethical-Review-and-the-Globalization-of-Clinical-T/ArticleStandard/Article/detail/83804.

CHAPTER 2

Transgenic Mosquitoes Project as Model

2.1 Introduction

A well-developed clinical trial protocol that is burning on all elements may be hard to find, but it doesn't have to. In *Guidance Framework for Testing of Genetically Modified Mosquitoes*[1] (hence forth to be called GMM report or GMM framework), the WHO has set an excellent example; one that is easily replicable.

Bent on tackling the widely-known pair of stubborn diseases, malaria and dengue fever, with a new age technology that enjoys a rich vein of form, the GMM attempt is a gilt-edged opportunity for the WHO. The depth and breathe of its craft are immense. If modern clinical trials with humans were looking for a responsible model, they have one in this framework.

In this chapter, the GMM framework is the major source material used. More specifically, a bulk of space in this chapter will be used up to reflect on the relevant aspects of this astutely packaged health information. When other source materials are discussed, it will be as they relate to the GMM model. In time, my intention to heavily rely on its use will become obvious, including, how it sharply contrasts with the Nigeria-Pfizer clinical trial example discussed in Chapter 1. Ultimately, this GMM report takes the form of what I would recommend as a paragon of what responsibility in clinical trials really ought to be. I will argue that the steps it suggests should be standard practice for *all* clinical trial protocols particularly those that use human subjects and including those with both direct and indirect ecological implications. This persuasive argument presages the thesis for this book: re-conceptualizing clinical trials with the concept of African personhood.

---

1 Sponsored by the World Health Organization, *The 2014 WHO Guidance Framework for Testing of Genetically Modified Mosquitoes* compendium is the product of the meeting of the minds of some of the best experts in the field. However, not all aspects of this dense report will pertain to my discussion, hence I will be referencing only the parts that are relevant to my thesis. I am greatly indebted, and I pay special tribute to Paul B. Thompson (my research committee member) for providing this document for my use. After learning about my research work, Thompson, a member of the think tank that formulated the report, made it available to me early as it was still receiving reviews and comments prior to its publication.

 | DOI 10.1163/9789004366947_004

In the second half of the chapter, I will point out (with some personal sense of satisfaction) that the GMM approach apparently boosts, without intending to do so, two important issues that relate with this work. My inclination for ecocentrism; holism or interconnectedness; and the intrinsic value of the biosphere in ranked order of being, are all widely shared philosophical perspectives in African thought. This will become clearer in Chapter 4 which discusses personhood in African thought. I will also draw on Aldo Leopold's deliberation on land ethic and the 'biotic community' which strikingly differs with individualist deontology and individualist cum consequentialist positions that pervade much of Western thinking.[2]

Two, by calling to mind the intimate connection between environmental and human health, the GMM report hits at the heart of a long-nursed intuition of mine, to reunite bioethics (here via clinical trials) with its estranged sibling, environmental ethics. As it stands, few people today are aware that bioethics and environmental ethics were joined at the hip at birth in the 1970s. But soon after that emergence they pathed ways, each field appearing to have evolved an individuality of their own without maintaining overt affinity. I would argue that their genetic unity should always be apparent. Hacking back to the African philosophical context where holism reigns, it comes as no surprise that these two broad issues can be merged into what I will refer to as bio-eco-communalism (BEC).[3]

2.2 Some Preliminaries

To put in perspective the challenge malaria and dengue fever scourges present in recent times, a few statistics are in order before turning to the GMM model. According to WHO's 2013 figures, an estimated 3.4 billion people in 97 countries were at risk of malaria, of whom 1.2 billion were at high risk. In comparison, there were an estimated 207 million cases of malaria in 2012; and an estimated 627, 000 deaths (482, 000 children under five years of

2 Read more about "The Land Ethic." In *Environmental Ethics: An Anthology*, Andrew Light and Holmes Rolston, (eds.), Blackwell Publishers Ltd., 2003.

3 Credits go to Godfrey Tangwa's (2004) ingeniousness in smithing the original term 'eco-biocommunalism.' See, "Some African Reflections on Biomedical and Environmental Ethics." In Kwasi Wiredu (Ed.). *A Companion to African Philosophy* (Oxford: Blackwell Publishers), 387–395. There he fuses eco-ethics, environmental ethics, developmental ethics, medical ethics, and bioethics under one label. The nomenclature I formulate here though related, is however different.

age – 1, 300 children every day, or one child almost every minute); 90% of the total number of malaria-related deaths occurred in Africa. Between 2000 and 2012, the scale-up of interventions helped to reduce malaria incidence rates by 25% globally, and by 31% in the WHO African Region. The global malaria mortality rate was reduced by 42% during the same period, while the decrease in the WHO African Region was 49%.[4] In spite of the seeming progress, the abatement, though a remarkable suppression, seems to hold down the scourge only momentarily, while the scourge continues to gulp more funding resources.

International disbursements for malaria control rose from US$100 million in 2000 to US$1.94 billion in 2012 and US$1.97 billion in 2013. National government funding for malaria programs has also increased since 2004 but not at the same pace; the total for 2012 was US$522 million. The currently available funding is far below the resources required to reach universal coverage of interventions. The WHO estimates that US$5.1 billion is needed every year for this purpose. In 2012, the global total of international and domestic funding for malaria was US$2.5 billion – less than half of what is needed.[5]

On its part, dengue is reportedly the most common mosquito-borne viral disease of humans that in recent years has become a major international public health concern. Globally, 2.5 billion people live in areas where dengue viruses can be transmitted. The geographical spread has led to the global resurgence of epidemic dengue fever and emergence of dengue hemorrhagic fever in the past 25 years with the development of hyperendemicity in many urban centers of the tropics. Dengue ranks as one of the most important mosquito-borne viral disease in the world. In the last 50 years, incidence has increased 30-fold. An estimated 2.5 billion people live in over 100 endemic countries and areas where dengue viruses can be transmitted. Up to 50 million infections occur annually with about 500, 000 cases of dengue hemorrhagic fever and 22,000 deaths mainly occurring among children.[6]

Both malaria and dengue are vector-borne diseases, meaning, diseases that are transmitted via a carrier or transporter. Mosquitoes are the agents of transportation that convey pathogens for these diseases into the host cells (for example, humans or birds). The GMM report has noted that mosquitoes

4 Information was culled from the *World Health Organization* "Factsheet on the World Malaria Report 2013," http://www.who.int/malaria/media/world_malaria_report_2013/en/. Viewed on May 28, 2014.

5 Ibid.

6 Read more at *World Health Organization*, "Dengue/Dengue Haemorrhagic Fever," http://www.who.int/csr/disease/dengue/en/. Viewed on May 28, 2014.

transmit several diseases of major global public health importance, but it focuses mainly on malaria and dengue fever.

It is against this backdrop; and owing to the intensified practice of transnational biomedical research; plus, the considerable controversy about the ethics of research, (see Chapter 1), that the GMM report could not have come at a better time. In that preceding chapter, I noted as well the enticing potential for exploitative tendencies for economic gains associated with some clinical trials, etc. To the contrary, the expectation is how ethical principles and community engagement, not profit motives, etc., should guide actions in determining how the cultural milieus of patient-subjects and residents of research sites must be engaged, respected, adequately compensated, and if possible, made to benefit from research outcomes. The urgent desire for further and continuing retooling of international guidelines or codes of research ethics and the considerable stakes involved also make the GMM guidance framework most timely. Approaches such as this, has long been recognized to underpin, "claims that, in addition to the direct benefits for individuals within the study, benefits should include the linkage of otherwise unavailable health care to research projects, provision of proven treatments following completion of trials, as well as community empowerment."[7]

For a quick comparison, I see a semblance of sorts between the GMM framework and a working paper that emerged in the early 1990s from a symposium on ethics and public health which examined the challenges of trans-cultural clinical malaria research in the developing world. While highlighting the need that such investigative collaboration requires a unique bridging of cultural differences with respect to human subject investigation, the setting addressed other germane issues. They include the difficulties of informed consent in different cultural settings; whether there is any role for community involvement; whether drug and vaccine trials not approved in an industrialized country are ever defensible if performed in an industrializing country; potential conflicting priorities between investigators; and, issues regarding conflict resolution.[8] Though commendable as stated, the tackling of these issues don't come close to the full-throated manner the GMM report formulates all the substantive

7 Benatar, Solomon. 2004. "Rationally Defensible Standards for Research in Developing Countries." *Health and Human Rights*, 8, 1: 197–202. A review of Ruth Macklin's book, *Double Standards in Medical Research in Developing Countries*.

8 Barry, Michele and Molyneux, Malcolm. 1992. "Ethical Dilemmas in Malaria Drug and Vaccine trials: A Bioethical Perspective." *Journal of Medical Ethics*, 18: 189–192. The symposium was sponsored by the Institute of Medicine and The American Society of Tropical Medicine and Hygiene.

and procedural aspects of the issues involved. Moreover, while the symposium analysis asks, for instance, whether or not there is a role for community involvement, the GMM framework provides a convincing logic why there should be, while pointing out the flaws in the mainstream informed consent process, etc. Altogether, the comprehensive footnotes and illuminating cross-references reflect the consummate knowledge of the multidisciplinary areas experts in the GMM project represent.

2.3 The GMM Model

Considering the adage that prevention is always better, I view the WHO's effort as a preventionist approach. It is a strategy built on attacking mosquito vectors *ab initio*, a method known to be one of the most effective ways to reduce transmission of diseases in endemic areas. This thinking accounted for the successful elimination of malaria transmission in parts of Europe and the U.S. at the turn of the 20th century, as well as stemming the spread of dengue fever in the Americas in the early 1960's. Moreover, it has been widely observed that the more prevalent method of relying on insecticides for vector control increases, rather than diminish, actually increases the risk that mosquitoes will develop resistance.[9]

Irked by the menacingly high death tolls in spite of control efforts amidst depleting funding resources, the WHO guidance framework aims to perfect a mechanism with the aid of molecular biology to develop genetically modified mosquitoes as an efficient public health tool to halt the transmission of malaria and dengue fever.[10] Due to its innovative, potent and more cost-effective approach, it is adjudged to trump other comparable methods such as radiation- and chemo-sterilization. Nonetheless, and specifically for reasons not to leave anything to chance, the multidisciplinary think tank behind this report (with expertise in molecular biology, medical entomology, ecological, legal, ethical, social and cultural areas) insists on the need for "thorough, thoughtful and transparent preparation for, and conduct of field trials of the GMM technology." The experts reiterate that the GMM method hints at providing a reliable model for all countries to emulate.

In a nut shell, the mechanics of the technology works when lab-hatched genetically modified mosquitoes are,

9 WHO GMM, p. xi.

10 Ibid, p. xi.

> ... made sterile and thus unable to pass the genetic modification on to future generations through mating. In other cases, the GMM are meant to mate and introduce the effect briefly into the local mosquito population, but the modification will gradually be diluted out by crossing with local mosquitoes over a number of generations until it is lost.[11]

The research experts were duly aware that in any novel method, some unknown outcomes could mean the possibility that this could take on a different trajectory outside of its intended purpose, potentially engendering among other things, grave ethical, environmental, social and other concerns. In light of this, they met at intervals over an extended period, debated, and fine-tuned implementation strategies for the testing of the genetically modified vectors. The result was the following broadly formulated two-tenet agreements which became their guide:

- First, field testing should begin with release of sterile or otherwise self-limiting modified male mosquitoes in order to gain experience with the technology under circumstances where its effects can be reversed by halting releases.
- Second, testing of modified mosquitoes incorporating gene drive should begin under physical confinement. No genetically-modified mosquitoes designed to replicate and spread the modification to wild-type mosquitoes [should be] tested outside of the laboratory.[12]

These assurances are bound to further boost confidence in the approach as it strives to foster quality and consistency in the processes for testing and regulating new genetic technologies.

Intense calls for ethics and public engagement in public health research is a claim that is often made, and the GMM report seems to underscore its importance to the hilt:

> Public dialog and outreach are important for realizing research goals, especially in the development of new technologies. Sincere and well-developed engagement can help to direct technical goals, reduce the chance of a misunderstanding of the science needed to meet the goals, and improve the performance of the research project in both technical and social contexts. Although engagement activities may overlap with

11 Ibid.

12 Ibid, p. xi.

> regulatory requirements, researchers should not assume that regulatory compliance also implies that ethical and engagement responsibilities have been adequately addressed. Respect for communities should be an overarching ethical goal in GMM trials.[13]

So crucial and integral are ethics and engagement efforts that it was urged that they be initiated early and at intervals throughout the study (and even after). Rightly noted, the role of ethics and engagement becomes crystal clear in the way that tensions are doused between scientists who are absorbed in the quest to realize the envisioned results of their research, and some in the public who view them as lacking in moral sensibility or fellow-feeling. Primed to be a 4-phased trial, the GMM report recommends that engagement activities be introduced during Phases 1 and 2,[14] to ensure that the goals and methods of the project are well defined and communicated to meet genuine stakeholder needs. I would rather suggest that considerations for ethics and engagement activities should commence at the planning stage (long before Phase 1). The advantage of this early application is to test the waters, meet with third party (outside) groups and individuals, and gauge the strategies in order to tweak any areas that might need improvements. It is at this stage that the GMM acknowledgment makes complete sense: engagement and involvement with the communities hosting the GMM trials must be guided by detailed knowledge of the local community, its institutions and common practices. Finding out what kinds of concerns the community might have, any past engagements around science that went badly, or determining what the community wants/expects in terms of engagement or consent [and assent] will be important. I also would suggest that it should outlast the research study at certain intervals until it fades out.

Field researchers stand to benefit when community engagement activities are expanded in Phase 3 specifically because they address ethical responsibilities beyond the formal permissions required at the individual level (informed consent/assent) and the governmental level (regulatory compliance). If it hasn't been made apparent already, meaningful engagement with the community, among other related actions, smoothens the path to obtaining authorization to conduct study. It states that the concept of 'community authorization' entails providing those living in the trial site with methods to give or withhold agreement for trial activities, and to identify elements they believe to be important for the research to continue. During field testing, scientists also should

13 Ibid, p. xv.

14 Ibid, p. 70.

expect to interact with third parties who express interest in the activity and its outcomes, both to ensure that the project is well understood and to avail the project team of information and insights that such interested parties might provide.[15] With tenacity and goodwill, by Phase 4, all stake holders would have gained deep appreciation of the research procedure to the point that the responsibilities for implementing the technologies being tested and interacting with affected individuals likely will shift to the relevant local, regional or national public health authorities.

Thus, the scope of ethical responsibilities and community engagement becomes the overarching goal in any project similar to the GMM project. My preference for engaging the community early on for greater understanding of purpose and successful project undertaking is supported by the idea that it would afford trial studies the opportunity to become aware of a laundry list of important issues likely to affect the study. For instance, John Olin, et al., identified factors that either motivate individuals to volunteer for a vaccine trial or disincentivize them to participate, along with preparedness of the larger community for trials. "Personal concerns for health and for the impact of the epidemic on families and country were common motivations for participation. The danger of an experimental vaccine and the stigma of a positive HIV antibody test as the result of vaccination are major concerns and disincentives. The health, educational, and local non-governmental sectors are identified as having important roles to play in assuring [community] preparedness for trials."[16]

The larger philosophical point that the GMM proposal precisely advocates is that ethics of engagement aims to identify and recognize the interests of stakeholders and their legitimate entitlements, rights, other types of claims and obligations, including what actions or activities that are necessary by the principle of respect for communities hosting the trials. As such, it brings into focus, such ethical issues as: how these rights and interests should be recognized in a decision for trials to proceed; how researchers can strike an ethically robust balance between the interests and rights of individuals, the collective interests of the host communities and the properly mandated activities of their public institutions; and, determining the appropriate role for communication and engagement with media, civil society organizations and others that take an interest in the research.[17]

15 Ibid, p. 59.

16 Olin, John. 2006. "Community Preparedness for HIV Vaccine Trials in the Democratic Republic of Congo" *Culture, Health & Sexuality*, 8, 6: 529.

17 WHO GMM report, p. 60.

Even on an individual level, the importance of ordinary word of mouth is highly rated particularly in how it can effectively disseminate a widely-shared impression of research goals, intended applications and methods, including within village, sub-urban, or city settings. Such broad representations of science can have the beneficial effect of expanding opportunities to obtain key informants, participants and partners. But if the community does not buy into it, the opposite effect will likely result, and that can include widespread misrepresentation, suspicion, distrust and even outright blackmail and antagonism against the scientific research project.

The GMM ethics and community engagement approach, like some of the concepts I have discussed here, also take the form of a concentric relational web: from the core research site/human research subjects, to their friends, families, and the larger community. The outer spectrum recognizes individuals who do not typically fall within the definition of human subjects but who might be affected by the conduct of research, either because they reside near the research project site, or that their daily activities and/or livelihood, including economic interests, could be affected by the research activities.

The GMM report remarks that on the other hand, people living at a distance from the trial site and are unlikely to be physically affected by the trial activities themselves, might still stake a very strong interest in the conduct or outcome of research simply because their interests overlap with those of their friends and relatives at the trial site. For instance, people who are under certain health conditions (and/or their friends and family) would likely have an obvious interest in the outcome of research or clinical trials, even if they are not involved with that specific trial. It adds that such groups are likely to be strongly supportive of research intended to improve their condition. Similarly, people who care about causes such as protecting vulnerable groups or endangered species are likely to take an interest in a wide range of research activities, and may as well be supportive of certain research goals or procedures.

Although the nature of responsibilities to such individuals or groups, the report says, is quite different from those of the research subjects and communities hosting the trial, it is clear that an effective plan for engaging a wide scale of such interested parties can be critical to the success of research, especially for projects that can possibly draw a significant public media attention or monitoring from civil society organizations. In this way, the onus of ethical responsibilities by researchers can be quite encompassing and even complicated, and meeting these responsibilities requires adequate preparation which can go a long way to smoothen rough edges by addressing the full range of stakeholder interests.

The GMM report provides a long list of such interested parties which include, persons associated with global or regional public health and international development organizations such as, governments; scientists and members of scientific organizations with disciplinary or inter-disciplinary links to research activities associated with field testing activities, including sciences dedicated to public health and infectious disease. Others are, persons and organizations engaged in competing approaches to control of infectious diseases; environmental and human rights activists. There is the added point to draw from the experience of GM crops to illustrate "the need also to consider possibilities for longer range economic, spiritual or cultural effects" scientific trials can have, and in what ways.[18]

Ordinarily, these are not the sorts of circumstances or communication apparati (and there are more to come) standard research budgets accommodate as far as most scientific studies are conceived and conducted. However, many scientists often view their work as having value and a social purpose, and this may be especially so for those conducting research on public health and disease control. But as the GMM report seems to indicate, the problem is that scientists are often not very transparent (particularly given the new global dispensation, plus the issue of private interest involvement in clinical trials, see Chapter 1). Also, many scientists do not always articulate the purpose of their research explicitly, or discuss its value with the public. The GMM guidelines certainly seeks to make explicit the value and social purpose of the scientific research project and suggests a broader reflection that serves several key functions and interests.[19]

John Ziman has made that ethical burden more categorical as scientists are having to perform new roles in which ethical considerations can no longer be swept aside as their products become more tightly woven into the social fabric.[20] This beam of thought is likewise reflected in Kevin Elliot's[21] discussion of "Ethics for Experts" or ethics of expertise, EOE. There, he develops a set of guidelines to assist researchers in sharing their study plans and findings; a move that will in turn assist the citizens, activists and policy makers as well to, for instance, enable them to better understand the societal ramifications of the research they do.

18 See, Ibid, pp. 67 & 72.

19 Ibid, p. 66.

20 Ziman, John. 1998. "Why Must Scientists Become More Ethically Sensitive Than They used to be?" Essays on Science and Society, *Science*, 282, 4.

21 Elliot, Kevin. 2011. *Is a Little Pollution Good for You?* New York: Oxford University Press, p. 133.

In particular, it is noted that hitherto, there was a lack of appetite in developing EOE for researchers even as the complexity involved in disseminating scientific findings to the public demands it. More so, the "scientists' social responsibilities in general (not to mention their specific responsibilities for disseminating information) have received less analysis than ethical issues internal to scientific practice (e.g., management of data, relationship among researchers, treatment of human and animal research subjects)."[22]

Thus far, there are enough grounds to be persuaded by the argument about the saliency of ethics and community authorization/engagement. But I want to make clear that it merely prepares the ground for other ethical requirements which are expressed in the informed consent/assent process. As I indicated in Chapter 1 (to be discussed further in Chapter 4), one of the major shortcomings of principlism is the lack of recognition that all research, directly or otherwise, do affect the larger communities and not just the individual study subjects (in fact, in most non-Western or communitarian cultures, every research, just like all social activities, is considered to have either direct or indirect effects on the community and/or environment, etc.). Likewise, the GMM guidelines have accurately highlighted the apparent implications particularly because the effects of the trials will largely be at the community level as well as on the environment.

2.4 GMM Model and Biodiversity

I turn to the GMM recommendations as they relate to the connection between human and environmental health. As I have already shown, it is with delight that I encounter this factual rarity (particularly in Western literature) that fuses human health and environmental health. To be fair, pioneers of the larger bioethics project built their vision on that unity of purpose before the field witnessed the current splinterization. But more importantly, it is a widely shared philosophical perspective, for instance, in Africa which recognizes the holism or interconnectedness and the intrinsic value of the biosphere in ranked order of being.

My point here is simply to give readers a picture of some of the reasons a researcher on a clinical trials mission might find the prospect of considering the safety of the environment appealing and as an integral part of their work. In certain clinical trial cases (e.g., the GMM trial) the connection is obvious, in others (e.g., the Trovan trial, see Chapter 1), it might be subliminal. Here,

22 Ibid: 135.

the GMM recommendation gets at the point by way of *biosafety*. The guidelines highlight the connection and hence proffer plans to address the safe use of technologies through the management of risks to the environment and to human health.[23]

The design of this public health intervention tool seriously considers the need to target the pathogens in a way that does not harm either environmental or human health (and non-human animals, etc.,). It recommends that the overarching ethical goal should be to respond to obligations to individuals being asked to participate as human research subjects and/or to communities being asked to host trials; while maintaining transparent and respectful channel of communication throughout and long after the trial period.

The key word here is *risk* which is defined as the combination of the magnitude of the consequences of a hazard (an unwanted event), if it occurs, and the likelihood that the consequences occur.[24] And the aim is how to avoid it if possible, or limit it as much as possible, and manage it to acceptable levels, if and when a hazard results. This is done through risk analysis, which when teased out gives rise to risk concern, risk assessment, risk management and risk communication. It explicates risk concern to mean alertness to and reason to worry about issues pertaining to both technology and social values, and in both cases supported evidence that a concern is valid. For risk assessment and management, the development of risk frameworks is necessary whereby qualitative, and where possible, quantitative pieces of evidence are used to assess the probability that an adverse event (a hazard) will occur and the consequences associated with the occurrence of that event. In essence, a risk analysis procedure accounts for the possibility of an event happening but which may or may not be harmful in particular circumstances. Ultimately, effective risk management can render many risks acceptable and manageable.[25] Per the WHO framework, biosafety risk assessment aims to determine,

> (i) the potential hazards and the mechanisms of impact for GMM on wild populations of target and non-target organisms; (ii) the likelihood and magnitude of impact of the GMM on the receiving environment; (iii) the levels and consequences of uncertainty associated with the effects, and (iv) appropriate risk management measures needed to mitigate any harm or uncertainty associated with changes to target organism populations or the wider receiving environments. Risk communication ensures that

23 Ibid, p. 33.

24 Ibid, p. 34.

25 Ibid, p. 33.

> there is a well-documented explanation of what risks have been identified, how they have been assessed, what the acceptable level of risk is, and how risk management may be able to achieve acceptable levels of risk with implementation.[26]

Just like the ethics and community engagement approach, biosafety measures are phased in with the different stages of the trial protocol during which specific possible hazards are addressed at their respective appropriate stages – from laboratory and cage environments to open field releases. In this way further testing stages that follow are made more workable and the protocol becomes better defined as appropriate decisions are reached. With respect to the GMM project, possible relevant hazards that might occur are covered in the following questions: Will release of the GMM increase transmission of the target or other diseases? Will release of the GMM cause a significant biting nuisance? And, will release of the GMM result in disruption to valued ecosystem components?[27]

It is apparent that estimating the degree of ecological risk from the introduction of a new technology such as GMM, involves an admixture of ethics, culture, science, economics and health. As noted already, the complexity can be illustrated by the experience of genetically engineered crops. An instance that helps to underline this abstruseness in the GMM project is the locomotive capabilities of mosquitoes. The report simply confirms what we have long known about mosquitoes that they make unpredictable movements between locations, in which case, it will be impossible, in advance, to say for sure all persons (or non-human animals) with whom they make contact. Moreover, knowledge from vector biology research had previously proposed that biosafety oversight may be a more appropriate model than individual human subject protection. Equally useful would be to apply lessons from other environmental health programs, which typically involve unavoidable risks and as such not amenable to ethical procedures that presume an opportunity to exit or opt out of the risk bearing situation.

In releasing transgenic mosquitoes into a designated site, it was hypothesized that some of the key consequences will likely be the alteration of ecosystem functions (such as role of mosquito larvae in the food chain for predators) and other impacts on target organisms through destabilization of local mosquito populations. The possibility of this unintended reality may pose a risk, according to the Guideline, particularly to human health if the GMM vector

26 Ibid, p. 33.

27 Ibid, p. 34.

control system fails after a release program is well advanced. "This might include assessing local mosquito populations for the evolution of resistance to the transgene function, the evolution of the disease pathogen to resist transgene function or changes in host range of targeted mosquito species."[28] It notes further the possibility of resurgence of disease when immunologically naïve human populations are exposed to disease after a prolonged period of low incidence as a concern that should be assessed in post-implementation monitoring. However, this is not unique to GMMs.

To itemize specifics, the ecological consequences that might occur, as identified by the GMM report, include,

- Effects on biological diversity
- Vertical gene transfer
- Horizontal gene transfer
- Persistence of the transgene in the ecosystem
- Evolutionary responses (especially in target mosquito vectors or pathogens)
- Unintentional trans-boundary movement (including international borders).[29]

The GMM literature therefore suggests that evolution and adaptive processes be considered and appropriate regulatory structures, mechanisms and methods need to be in place as integral parts of the risk assessment to ensure that clear lines of responsibility are delineated on post-implementation surveillance. In effect, post implementation monitoring should draw on evidence from earlier Phases to determine the need for and design of monitoring to observe the key impacts identified.

The Guideline report concludes that biosafety measures ought to be buoyed further by independent constituencies or review boards. This appears to fit with its promise of maintaining transparency and permitting of objectivity and candor.

All in all, the foregoing marks a shift from considering ethics of research within the bare bones of principlism, to considering the ethics of research in a much broader sense. The GMM model for biosafety, ethics of engagement, etc., reveal the need to improve the links between research and health care delivery and to promote the environmental, cultural, socio-political and economic processes that are involved so we can begin to widen our understanding of the

28 Ibid, pp. 49–50.

29 Ibid, p. 49.

vicissitudes of the impacts of public health research (or any other research for that matter).

After reviewing and analyzing 14 case studies and articles in 2006, Dianne Quigley came to somewhat similar conclusions. Her work focused on research ethics issues in the conduct of environmental and public health research with Native American and other indigenous populations. She highlighted how community-based participatory research practices can provide working guidelines that can overcome past research harms.[30]

As observed, the successful implementation of GMM interventions requires transparent, focused, proportionate and credible biosafety assessments. The significance of the role of stakeholder groups such as individual communities is evident as they provide the key to appropriately deal with the ethical and cultural dimensions. They should likewise provide consistent and strong voice within both biosafety and benefit-cost analyses associated with the testing and implementation of GMMs.[31]

I can understand if some curious observer thinks that the GMM model and traditional clinical trial model are like apples and oranges. However, I see more similarities than dissimilarities. Yes, the GMM model contains no typical human subjects. That is about the only major difference. But when we think comprehensively and holistically, the tunnel vision we've had will melt away and morph into a quick realization why the GMM recommendation extends to just about all clinical trials.

Couched within the philosophical commitment to evaluate clinical trials in terms of ecological and human health, the GMM project seems to necessitate a healthy debate. It does so while resolutely pursuing efficacy, transparency, responsible sense of purpose, quality and consistency in the process of testing and regulating new genetic technologies. After several decades of treating bioethics and environmental ethics as distinct disciplines, it appears that our collective capacity to understand and discuss them jointly need revamping. Bioethicists and environmental philosophers should hence forth take up the gauntlet to refocus on that discussion. That is the thrust of the next segment.

---

30 Details are in "A Review of Improved Ethical Practices in Environmental and Public Health Research: Case Examples from Native Communities." *Health Educational Behavior*, 33: 130.

31 Ibid, p. 51.

2.5 Environmental Ethics and Bioethics

It would be recalled that bioethics and environmental ethics were of the same allele which came to life simultaneously in the 1970s. Though identical off-shoots, they seem to have evolved in separate ways soon after. Since that feigned parting of ways each seem to maintain an individuality of their own without manifesting much of if any, overt affinity. How or why they appear to take on this posture may be a fair question. In fact, the opening salvo in the book, *The Ethics of Environmentally Responsible Health Care* by Jessica Pierce and Andrew Jameton (2004), laments that separation into what looked like irreconcilable paths even as both fields remain hinged on a common philosophical substratum: ethics.

A more cogent inquiry would be to ask, can they reconcile as they were originally conceived so as to address practical concerns that are common to them? For sure, the inspiration that the GMM framework presents already has given us a heads-up in that direction. Properly considered, environmental and human matters should not be separated from each other.

In 1970, when Van Porter used the term *bioethics*,[32] his concern went beyond the confines of medical ethics. He was troubled by the emerging global

32 Obviously, there is more than one account of how the term "bioethics" originated. Robert Martensen credits statesman Sargent Shriver, for coining the word "bioethics" in his own Bethesda, Maryland living room one night in 1970. It was at the instance of meeting with physician Andre´e Hellegers, a Jesuit philosopher and then president of Georgetown University and others, to discuss (President) Kennedy family sponsorship of an institute for the application of moral philosophy to concrete medical dilemmas. Martensen however cedes that Van Rensselaer Potter, "conceptualized bioethics expansively." Read more from Martensen's 2001, "The History of Bioethics: An Essay Review," *Journal of the History of Medicine and Allied Sciences*, 56, 2: 168–175. Dianne Irving on her part, locates the embryonic formation of "bioethics" in the 1960s following Congressional and Senate hearings which were called to "address an increasing number of knotty and bewildering problems especially being generated by medical research and the abuse of human subjects." See details in Irving's 2000 unpublished essay, "What is 'bioethics'? (*Quid est 'bioethics'?"*). However, the Internet Encyclopedia of Philosophy thinks that all the Above oft-cited stories might be incorrect. Crediting H.M. Sass' 2007 work, it states that indeed it was the German Theologian Fritz Jahr whose three published articles in 1927, 1928, and 1934, that first used the German term "Bio-Ethik" (which translates as "Bio-Ethics"). From then on, a new academic discipline was established, and gradually the commencement of "the practice of a new, more civilized, ethical approach to issues concerning human beings and the environment. Jahr famously proclaimed his bioethical imperative: 'Respect every living being, in principle, as an end in itself and treat it accordingly wherever it is possible.'"

environmental crisis and the challenges of the earth's survival. That explains why, two decades later, he reframed it as *global bioethics*, to accurately reflect his thinking and foster a re-conceptualization of an ethics of health care as it relates to Earth care and global survival. Porter, an oncologist, saw a constant thread of unity whether it was in his cancer research or any other aspect of life and concluded that much of mankind's problems were our inability to forge a synergy between the two broad cultures of science and the humanities. "Ethical values cannot be separated from biological facts. We are in great need of a Land Ethic, a Wildlife Ethic, a Population Ethic, a Consumption Ethic, an Urban Ethic, an International Ethic, a Geriatric Ethic, and so on."[33]

To the extent that we have endured this disconnect for too long presses the need for the immediate bridging of medical and ecological ethics, recognizing them as one and their critical role in the future of health and environmental planning for all species, human and non-human. Peter Whitehouse draws directly from Van Potter's original intuition to characterize the syndrome and to recommend a treatment plan. The bridging effort should be seen as the most expansive aspiration that contributes to the "development of viable programs of sustainable medicines in a sustainable environment."[34]

The work of Jessica Pierce and Andrew Jameton[35] seems exactly primed to achieve that aim. It maintains that high quality, ethically sound health care is

---

33 Potter, 1971. *Bioethics: Bridge to the Future*. Englewood Cliffs, New Jersey: Prentice-Hall, Inc. There is little wonder why he dedicated this work to the memory of Aldo Leopold who he says anticipated the extension of ethics to bioethics. More of van Potter's exegesis on this subject matter are available in the following publications: *Global Bioethics: Building on the Leopold Legacy*. East Lansing Michigan: Michigan State University Press, 1988; "Getting to the Year 3000: Can Global Bioethics Overcome Evolution's Fatal Flaw?" *Perspectives in Biology and Medicine*, 34, 1:89–98, 1990; Potter, Van and Potter, Lisa. 1995. "Forum: Global Bioethics: Converting Sustainable Development to Global Survival." *Medicine and Global Survival*, 2, 3:185–191; Porter, Van and Whitehouse, Peter. 1998. "Deep and Global Bioethics for a Livable World." *The Scientist*, 12: 9; and, "Fragmented Ethics and 'Bridges Bioethics.'" *Hastings Center Report* 29, 1:38–40, 1999.

34 Whitehouse, Peter. 1999. "The Ecomedical Disconnection Syndrome." *The Hastings Center Report*, 29, 1: 41.

35 Pierce, Jessica and Jameton, Andrew. 2004. *The Ethics of Environmentally Responsible Health Care*. Oxford: Oxford University Press, p. vi. While I mostly agree with the authors, some of the explicit ideals they identify as underlying the moral principles of both fields fail by way of not accurately accounting for their supposed defining differences. For instance, they state that health-care ethics (read, bioethics) focus on individual patients and their care givers; environmental ethics deals in large populations; and that clinical ethics episodes are usually resolved in days and months, while ecological issues play out over decades and even millennia. Many concrete bioethical instances don't bear these

guaranteed to be available, if and only if the larger environment is robustly viable enough to sustain good health.

It all seems so intuitive, yet we are reminded that we cannot, in our constant quest for specialization, continue to compartmentalize our daily lives, our health and wellbeing, from reality even as the myriad elements in the ecosystem that are interdependent on each other in the web of life. From microorganisms and tiny entomological species to large mammals, and the role each plays; from thinking about the safety of the water we drink to thinking about the quality of air we breathe. That we continue to simply insist that there is a distinction between environmental implications of our decisions and ethical judgments in health care and paying little attention to axiomatic philosophical action theory, seems a serious lapse in scholarly rigor. Genetic epidemiology has long proven that human diseases result from a combination of genetic inheritance and the environment and no other affirmation highlights the premise of that argument better.[36]

It is easy to discern why there is constant connection in everything. As an illustration, consider the long process in a drug or medical device production whereby biomedical scientists produce a medical device or cancer drug; IRB committees determine which of them meet clinical trial protocols – federal and state laws; and FDA decides when to approve for market-wide use. What is less known is how often, if at all, any of the actors involved has pondered over the ecological root cause or causes of the cancer disease that is being targeted. But a WHO study, as an example, may have put paid to that disconnection just as Porter envisioned. Data for the WHO finding established that 223,000 deaths from lung cancer around the world were caused by air pollution in 2013.

The International Agency for Research on Cancer, a branch of the WHO that did the study, now classifies air pollution in the same category as tobacco smoke, UV radiation and plutonium. And although air pollution had been known to cause heart and lung diseases, latest evidence provides additional data supporting the fact it also was causing different forms of cancer.[37]

---

claims out. True, some bioethical issues might be short-term, but most outlast generations. And yes, some also deal with individual patients but most deal with very large populations too. In essence, the authors' argument for a more integration of the two fields would be made stronger if they recognize that defining similarities are far greater, and that differences (between bioethics and environmental ethics) are far fewer than they have articulated.

36 Khoury, Muin. 1997. "Genetic Epidemiology and the Future of Disease Prevention and Public Health." *Epidemiology Reviews*, 19, 1:176.

37 WHO: International Agency for Research on Cancer, Press Release, No. 221, October 17, 2013.

Questions that Pierce and Jameton pose and the compelling answers they proffer to prove their point are poignant. Their core questions include, what concepts from environmental ethics can be applied to health care and how can they be combined with more traditional health-care ethics concepts? What kinds of case studies in health care highlight both clinical and environmental principles? Ultimately, they are of the view that environmental principles are the pivot of a responsible inclusive understanding of bioethics and conduct of health care (and probably, vice-versa).[38]

Further still, prescriptions in the GMM report regarding ecological health could have been informed by sentiments akin to the ones echoed in the complex theory of environmental responsibility that Akadémiai Kiadó[39] developed. In its broadest form, Kiadó's theory covers such areas as political, bioethical, scientific, and economic systems. Its emphasis on environmental protection is palpable in the way it simultaneously applies numerous systems of responsibility. "The whole theory of environmental responsibility is impregnated by the ubiquitous natural and civilizational responsibilities (borne by humans), whose presence and proportions determine both the quality and quantity of responsibility for the environment. In brief, the theory of complex environmental responsibility not only extends theoretical science, but also promotes orientation in the practice of environmental protection. It may be regarded as a new means of interpretation, though its main goal is to promote the practice of environmental protection."[40]

There is a moral burden in maintaining this order or else, the positive relation between individuals and between humans and the natural ecosystem will be negatively impacted. In tune with typical African philosophy and traditional belief, nature (reality) is an organic whole, and the creation and sustenance of ecological balance or interdependence between human and non-humans, the visible and the invisible are most desired. This in other words, points to holistic perspective (an emphasis on the interrelatedness or interconnectedness of everything in nature), as opposed to Western anthropocentrism (a social paradigm that values nature instrumentally and in so doing maintains the isolation of humans from nature and only sees its usefulness to humans).

One influential view that seemed to differ from this was that of *John Muir*, the Scottish-American naturalist and early advocate of preservation of wilderness in the U.S. While he believed in the intrinsic value and rights of all creatures

---

38 Ibid.

39 Kiadó, Akadémiai. 2011. "Theory of Complex Environmental Responsibility." *Társadalomkutatás*, 29, 3: 303–314.

40 Ibid.

and that a divine spirit flows in nature; he equally "valued nature for the sake of scientific research, for recreation, aesthetic enjoyment and spiritual inspiration,"[41] an attribute that didn't quite distinguish him just like most of his 19th century contemporary preservationists in America. However, one pre-eminent 19th century perspective – that of Aldo Leopold's – seems to hit the point well out of the ball park. In advocating a "land ethic" – the view that our moral concern should cover the natural environment and its nonhuman contents – he inspired several thinkers to advance the idea for "moral obligations toward ecological wholes, such as species, communities, and ecosystems, not just their individual constituents."[42] At Leopold's urging the argument goes that individual interests and well-being should be subsumed under the holistic good of the earth's biotic community.[43] Hence his famous line:

> That land as a community is the basic concept of ecology, but that land is to be loved and respected is an extension of ethics… A thing is right when it tends to preserve the integrity, stability, and beauty of the biotic community. It is wrong when it tends otherwise.[44]

With that, I segue into the more expansive African philosophical point of view about which Workineh Kelbessa illuminates with the Oromo ecotheology which teaches a positive relationship between the environment, humanity and their deity. I could have used any ethnic group anywhere on the African continent to make this point, but Kelbessa's research of the world view of the Oromo ethnic group, the largest in Ethiopia, is representative of a typical perspective that can easily be replicated across Africa. All African communities, with a varying wealth of symbolism, have analogous interpretations.

> There is a positive relationship between God and the Earth, humans and the natural environment. All creatures are essentially effected and affected by the harmonious relationship between Waaqa and the Earth. Waqaa is the creator of various creatures and is responsible for their existence. He requires humans to responsibly cohabit the Earth with other creatures…

41 Cited in Kelbessa, Workineh. 2011. *Indigenous and Modern Environmental Ethics*. Washington DC: Cultural Heritage and Contemporary Change, Series II, Africa, 13: 51.

42 *Stanford Encyclopedia of Philosophy*, "Environmental Ethics," http://plato.stanford.edu/entries/ethics-environmental/. Viewed on June 20, 2014.

43 Ibid.

44 Leopold, Waldo. 1949. *A Sand County Almanac*, Oxford: Oxford University Press, pp. vii–ix, 224–225.

For the Oromo, the land is not simply property to be exploited by humans without due respect and care. It is intrinsically valuable and requires respect and protection on the part of its inhabitants. If humans continuously despoil the land by breaking traditional rules and the cosmic purpose, it may not support all creatures indefinitely. The Oromo believe that the present generation has responsibility to pass on natural resources in good order to a future generation. That is why the Oromo are concerned with the health and peace of the environment and its inhabitants. They depend on environmental resources to heal themselves.[45]

The point seems to be that the continued neglect of this philosophical perspective in favor exclusively of anthropocentrism, is the bane of much of human crisis. For instance, a review paper by Richard Ingwe, Joseph Ebegbulem and C. Ikeji has tried to link anthropocentric policies and crises in climate/environment, finance and economy (especially by advanced economies) to the complete neglect of ecocentric world view as it pertains to contemporary African situation. "Specifically, pursuing the objectives, goals and interests of human beings without considering ecological principles or the inter-relatedness of human and non-human natural systems is responsible for the climate-environmental crisis."[46]

They recommend a back-to-the roots solution whereby think-tanks are formed to refocus and reinstitute various disciplines in the nexus of the development of both human and non-human natural environmental systems.

In smithing the word "eco-bio-communitarianism" Godfrey Tangwa, a pioneer and influential theorist who has blazed a trail in philosophical discussions on environmental ethics from an African point of view, attempts to strike some balance. While preferring eco-bio-communal outlook over anthropocentric ethic, Tangwa however concedes it doesn't necessarily mean it is an end-all panacea to all health and environmental problems. Nonetheless, he thinks it is a better option that is guaranteed to abate the urgent global hazards which have arguably been traced to anthropocentrism: "myriad problems

45 Kelbessa, Workineh. 2011. *Indigenous and Modern Environmental Ethics: A Study of the Indigenous Oromo Environmental Ethic and Modern Issues of Environment and Development*, Washington DC: Cultural Heritage and Contemporary Change, Series II, Africa, Vol. 13, pp. 85–86. His other relevant works include, "Indigenous Environmental Philosophy." *The Oxford Handbook of World Philosophy*. Oxford: Oxford University Press, 2011; and, "The Utility of Ethical Dialogue for Marginalized Voices in Africa" [A discussion paper], 2005.

46 Ingwe, Richard; Ebegbulem, Joseph and Ikeji, C. 2010. "Ecocentric and Anthropocentric Policies and Crises in Climate/Environment, Finance and Economy: Implications of the Emerging Green Policy of the Obama Administration for Africa's Sustainable Development." *African Journal of Political Science and International Relations*. 4, 1: 1–012.

of global pollution (of air, water, and soil); global climate change; of massive risks to plants, animals, and humans from toxic industrial wastes and from sophisticated weapons (conventional, nuclear, chemical, and biological); risks of upsetting nature's ecological balance; risk of accidentally triggering the collapse of the very foundations of life via gene technology, etc."[47]

In case the reader hasn't yet noticed, I have applied holism and ecocentrism as synonymous terms. This is intentional particularly as they ease into my preferred nomenclature, bio-eco-communitarianism, BEC. There is the claim that in the last few decades, environmental ethics has become an inherently holistic pursuit in large part due to Aldo Leopold's earlier mentioned outstanding influence. Also, the rapid calls for its adoption in environmental ethics have assumed Doppler proportions each time the matter comes up for discussion.

Michael Nelson[48] delineates environmental ethical holism as "the position that moral significance attaches to wholes over and above the individuals they include, or the idea that environmental wholes can and do matter morally and directly, or that they possess intrinsic value … what we are pointing to or looking for … we are exploring or desiring a system that allows us to directly morally include species, ecosystems, watersheds, biotic communities, or entities we typically consider collectives."

Charles Verharen's three-pronged view of holism is equally illuminating. First, it is a claim that all reality constitutes a single being; then that it is a commitment to join together what has been split apart; and lastly, that it is a claim that a single principle binds all existence together.[49] While Aldo Leopold is probably modern time's most authoritative influence on those who propose holistic ethics, alas, very little (if any) credit has been attributed to the ancient African root of that philosophical orientation. Citing Cheikh Anta Diop, Verharen explains that most ancient Egyptian cosmologies attribute the origins of the universe to a single principle such as *Nun*, through a process of becoming out of an original chaotic matter (water). "Through that same creative process,

47 Tangwa, Godfrey. 2004. "Some African Reflections on Biomedical and Environmental Ethics." *A Companion to African Philosophy.* Kwasi Wiredu (Ed.), Oxford: Blackwell Publishers, p. 393.

48 For a helpful discussion on holism see "Teaching Holism in Environmental Ethics" an unpublished pedagogical paper by Michael Nelson, a professor of environmental ethics and philosophy with interests in wilderness, wolves, and wildlife ecology, 2010.

49 Verharen, Charles. 2006. "Philosophy against Empire: An Ancient Egyptian Renaissance." *Journal of Black Studies*, 36, 6: 960. This view point is however original to Don Marietta and espoused in his 1995 work, *For People and the Planet: Holism and Humanism in Environmental Ethics*, Philadelphia: Temple University Press.

Khepera, the basic physical elements come into being, and from those elements evolve the gods, humans, and the world as we know it." In essence, the ancient Egyptians joined spirit together with matter, in which case humans were not separate from animals and even gods. Hence, the ancient African progenitor inspired holistic philosophies that have exerted a powerful hold on human imagination.[50]

By some unintended way, I have come to think that globalization might shed off its negative image with the saving grace embedded in the ontological concept of African holism. For one, the immensely complex global economy (and everything else), have within the last 20-odd years, surged to integrate at a vortex, thanks to globalization. By the same token, the ultimate reduction of complexity to simplicity which is found in the philosophy of holism might just be the solution we need. Verharen seems to share the same vision, "Unlike the history of the universe [the Big Bang Theory], the history of thought has moved in the direction of simplicity, defined as the smallest number of symbols capable of describing the greatest range of experience." Consequently, he urges for a return to our roots. The roots of all humans, as the whole world is finally beginning to discover, are in Africa.[51] I agree.

To wrap up, I reference a recent call out of Southern Queensland, Australia – one of the few efforts resembling the African perspective – that aims to redirect our understanding of sustainable development to a more ecocentric reorientation. If this call from 'Down Under,' typifies the emerging picture in the Western bloc, it could be a sign that signals the shifting posture which adds impetus to the fact that ecocentrism (or BEC) could be catching on. It examines the limitations in the contemporary anthropocentric conceptualization of sustainable development with a utilitarian ethic and argues for a more ecocentric reinterpretation of its definition that is more inclusive and incorporates recognition of the socio-ecological values. That in practical terms, is a recourse to finding lasting global resolution and a framework for sustainable development based on a reinterpretation that recognizes the interdependence of humans with the rest of the ecosphere.[52]

---

50 Ibid, pp. 960–961. Molefi Asante reflects further on the contributions of ancient African philosophy in *The Egyptian Philosophers: Ancient African Voices from Imhotep to Akhenaten*, Chicago: African American Images.

51 Ibid, p. 961.

52 Imran, Sophia; Alam, Khorshed; and Beaumont, Narelle. 2014. "Reinterpreting the Definition of Sustainable Development for a More Ecocentric Reorientation." *Sustainable Development*. 22: 134–144.

2.6 Concluding Thoughts

This chapter has witnessed a rich constellation of ideas including a blaze-trailing clinical trial GMM protocol that threads together human and eco-centric environmental philosophy which origin I have traced all the way to the ancient African thought. As summarized in Figure 1, the GMM framework has unintentionally rendered a catalogue of services that fit perfectly with my thesis. (1) My over-arching aim to reconceive responsibility in clinical trials with comprehensive considerations for research subjects and family, community engagement, respect for culture, biosafety, etc. (2) By calling to mind the intimate connection, namely the inseparability between environmental and human health, the GMM report hits at the heart of a long-nursed intuition of mine, to bring together bioethics (here via clinical trials) with its lost sibling, environmental ethics. (3) The GMM's methodology buoys my inclination for eco-centrism; holism or interconnectedness; and the intrinsic value of the

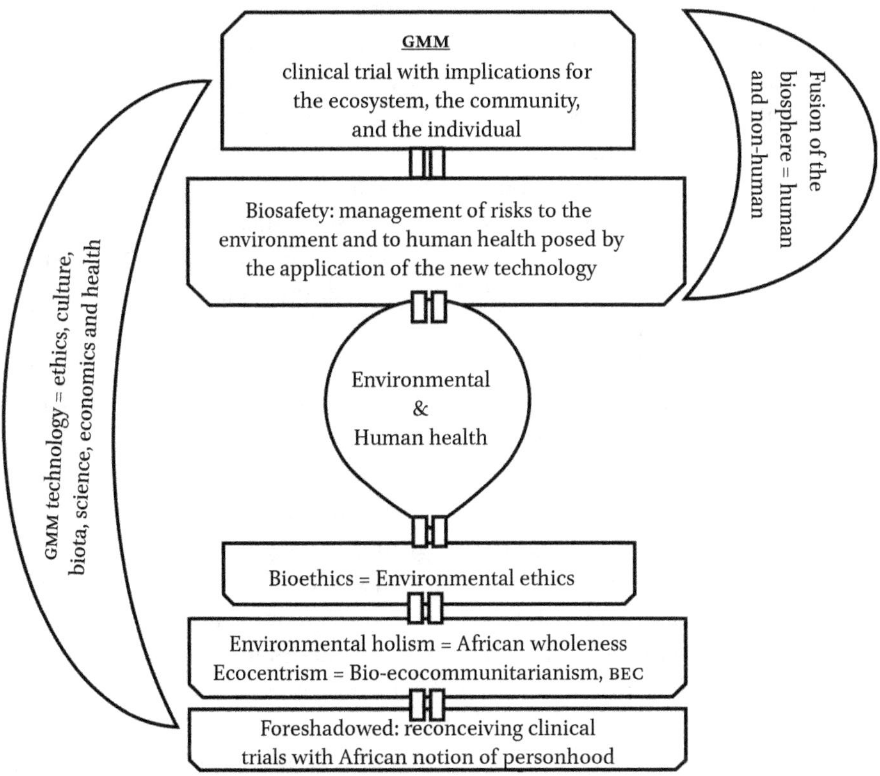

FIGURE 1 *Meeting of GMM framework, environmental/human health, and African holism.* FIGURE BY THE AUTHOR

biosphere in ranked order of being, which are widely shared philosophical perspectives in African thought.

(4) Even as the GMM protocol doesn't directly deal with human study subjects, nonetheless its approach is yet another indictment of sorts on the four principles of research ethics (principlism). It marks a shift from considering ethics of research solely within the bare bones of principlism to considering the ethics of research in a much broader sense. It engages the transgenic project in the fight against malaria and dengue fever as an all-encompassing endeavor; revealing the need to improve the links between environmental and human health, and to promote the cultural, socio-political and economic processes that are in-built.

Put together, this analysis benefited from relevant parts of that compendium to build a persuasive argument that presages the thesis for this book, namely a re-conceptualization of responsibility in clinical trials with the concept of African personhood (see Chapter 4).

From the outset, I tried to string together relevant aspects of the WHO's *Guidance framework for testing of genetically modified mosquitoes* which have collectively been the recurrent index for reflection. As a clinical trial protocol with an exceptional merit, I have argued that the steps it recommends should be standard practice for *all* clinical trial protocols including those that use human subjects and/or have ecological impact. For instance, this public health intervention tool lays out a well-developed ethical and engagement strategies by reducing the chance of misunderstanding the science needed to meet the goals, and improving the performance of the research project in both technical and social contexts. As such it made respect for individuals within communities the arrow head of its overarching ethical goal.

Then, for unusually melding human and environmental health – a move that bolsters the views of a section of the philosophy community (me included) that have pined for the urgent reconciliation of bioethics and environmental ethics – two areas (that should remain as one specialized field) with a fundamental basis for the pursuit of a common purpose. So fundamentally similar that they both share significant overlap on many issues – approaches, concepts, and moral considerations. That, in and of itself, extends to the ecocentric philosophical view point of holism or interconnectedness and the intrinsic value of the biospheral elements in ranked order of being. It comes as no surprise that these two broad issues can be merged into what I have referred to as BEC.

It is thus unprecedented that a clinical trial protocol with a Western origin has gone beyond the four-corners of principlism to recognize the possibility of a new technology (such as GMM), of having the potential to simultaneously impact human individuals, the community and the ecosystem in tandem. This fusion of elements in the biosphere (human and non-human) by implication makes a strong statement about the interrelatedness/interconnectedness of such factors as ethics, culture, the biota, science, economics and health (environmental and human). In so doing it has adequately positioned biosafety, namely the management of risks, as an integral point of consideration on issues relating to the environment and to human health as brought about by the application of the new technology.

In this same reasoning, if considerable attention is paid to the individual human subjects in clinical trials and how they exist only in reference to their community and the environment (the African notion), the import of my recommendation becomes crystal clear. Obviously, humans do not exist in a vacuum (forget the skewed emphasis on anthropocentrism). I suggest that while individualism and individual rights might be the primary concern for research ethics in the mainstream (Euro-American) practice, that and much more would be the case in research ethics at other places (such as Africa). And with more frequent off-shoring of biomedical studies, clinical investigators should pivot to BEC – an understanding that results from re-conceptualizing personhood within the context of communitarianism and eco-centrism. Details of this are in Chapter 4. But before we get to that, what do we know about the concept of responsibility? That is the concern of the next chapter where attempts will be made to present some answers.

PART 2

Responsibility

CHAPTER 3

Being Responsible

3.1 Introduction

Are you responsible? Should you be? Ought you? For whom; for what? For your livelihood, your wellbeing? For your two-year old son, Chukwuzita? For your 93-year old father, Anibeze? For licensing and vaccinating your dog? For your college loan? For your utility bills, your credit card debt, and your house mortgage? For acting to fix the rental car you damaged while 'drive-by-tweeting'? For the department or college, you are heading? For the military personnel in your platoon? For the safety of all passengers in the coach you are driving? For the young boy scouts in the summer camp you manage? For the players in the soccer team you coach? For the security of the nation you are leading? For the electorate, whose tax money pays your salary? For the public who rely on the auto products you make? For consumers of your farm produce? For the human subjects in your clinical studies? For a stranger under attack by a rabid canine? For donating to charity organizations (because of their good causes)?

The list is endless, but you get the idea. Consider this: it is not from the benevolence of the president, the governor or the legislator that we expect good governance, but from regard to their own political interest. But, even that interest is rooted in probity – responsibility. People generally act in conformity with the law, and in accordance with their individual morality as shaped by cultural and/or religious beliefs – all things being equal. Moreover, there are processes and procedures to be followed in governance. Deviate from that and you could be courting trouble.

The theme of this chapter is of course 'responsibility.' But I hasten to reassure the reader that this will not be a tortuous foray into the age-old philosophical debate on the concept of responsibility. In fact, let me apologize upfront for revisiting a philosophical concept that seem to have been thoroughly discussed through history. Nonetheless, my approach here promises a fresh breath on a concept so old it could belong to the antediluvian era. By this I recognize that 'responsibility' is both a simple and an extremely difficult, even contentious conceptual or theoretical theme that theorists have wrestled with from the dawn of time with some claiming to have long analyzed and reduced it to tiniest of parts and then coupled back.

 | DOI 10.1163/9789004366947_005

But regardless of the presumption that it has been critically threshed and winnowed out since the cradle of time, it however continues to challenge philosophers, neuroscientists and psychologists as they strive to understand what motivates human actions. In this book I don't have to reinvent the wheel, instead I make bold to present what could pass as an unorthodox, yet valid perspective overall to validate my mission to reconceive the term (responsibility). Thus, in my quest to provide a working perspective or delineation of the concept, I plan to make 'whistle-stop' mentioning of the relevant aspects of it – moral, legal, and so on – in a way that achieves my purpose.

This chapter contains three sections. In the first section, I will consider a select view of some schools of thought, historical references and/or explanations about the concept of responsibility (while avoiding a recast of worn out details). It is with such hindsight that the reader can appreciate the trajectory of my argument for a reconceptualization which will be introduced later in the project. This approach will hopefully supply the relevant substrate on which to hoist my new project.

The second section will deal with responsibility as a virtue. I will show how the virtue of responsibility can point to what it means to act responsibly[1] (a theme that will ultimately be tailored to fit the public health sector – clinical trials). I will resist to be drawn into the sea-saw argument (a common exercise in the literature) of whether or not we are responsible for our actions; to argue that living by a sense of responsibility can help to resolve issues that confront us on a day-to-day basis.

As a heads-up, the obligation to be responsible can at times be formal, i.e., codified as in traffic laws; or simply ingrained in the society's mores. In these instances, responsibility comes across as both a normative as well as a descriptive term. But besides the great emphasis on the normative side of responsibility, I wish to draw attention to the fact that it also ought to be conceived of in terms of a virtue. In presenting an account of the virtue of responsibility, I aim to add fillip to the reasoning that goes with both individual and collective responsibility.

In the third and final section, and given that the 1996 drug experimentation with some Nigerian children by Pfizer provided the stimulus for this research, it bodes well to devote some space – essentially join the fray – to address whether or not private enterprises and big corporations have other

1 It is almost impossible not to think of ancient historical foundations of virtue ethics which often connects with Plato, Aristotle but more accurately the pre-ancient African mysticism. But I will reference some recent works as well such as the one by Sabina Lovibond, 2002. *Ethical Formation*. Cambridge, Massachusetts: Harvard University Press.

responsibilities in addition to the responsibility to generate revenue for their owners and/or shareholders. In brief, I am opposed wholesale, to the argument that shields corporations from, for instance, social responsibility, merely on the claim that profit-making trumps everything else. Hence, I will claim that just as companies cannot engage in such questionable practices as polluting the environment with toxic chemicals, producing unsafe and lethal products, or lying and deceiving in advertising without adequate sanctions;[2] so too would, say, biomedical corporations not be left to their whims to engage in questionable practices but held to high standards of responsibility, including corporate social responsibility, CSR, when they conduct research with human subjects.

Hence, I will offer an explanation and defense for including corporations (as legal entities/persons) within the moral community. This is contained in my overarching project for the reconceptualization of the requirements for the rational application of responsibility, *à la* CSR. My approach will in turn address the objections by opponents of CSR.

My aim is not to satisfy these objectors. To the contrary, the burden of proof is upon them to show how contemporary enterprises could thrive without some reasonable measure of CSR. I contend that it is no longer possible to supply valid arguments to prove CSR morally irrelevant not withstanding that objectors continue to ignore the realities of action theory and pretend as if corporate actions and the social environments exist in parallel universes that never influence each other.

3.2 Understanding Responsibility

Certain things are easy to imagine however, most rational people will concede that no amount of "insight will render a society recognizable as a human society"[3] without some reasonable conception and appropriate application of responsibility. This in other words, is a tacit reminder that the core ingredients of acts of responsibility so conceived, are encoded in the genetic building blocks of all human systems, constituting their social life thereof.[4]

---

2 White, James. 1985. *Contemporary Moral Problems*. St. Paul Minnesota: West Publishing Company.

3 See David Risser's analysis of "Collective Moral Responsibility" on the *Internet Encyclopedia of Philosophy*. Accessed at http://www.iep.utm.edu/virtue/ on April 09, 2014.

4 For more, read Robert Hinde's "Responsibility: A Biological Perspective." There he establishes how the evolution of social behavior is rooted in many aspects of moral codes that are based in human psychological predispositions which in turn, have become codified in the course

The dictionary meaning of responsibility refers to the quality or state of being responsible as in, moral, legal, social or mental accountability.[5] At the rudimentary level that most people agree with, responsibility is a term that describes activities in situations involving moral agents or entities on a day-to-day basis. In particular, it suggests as well as assumes a form of obligation or duty (moral, social, legal, etc.) which we owe to ourselves, to others, to non-human animals, to the society and/or the environment within a given circumstance. Not uncommonly, we are won't to recognize such compelling accounts as this one by Gustafson and Laney.[6]

> Structures of mutual responsibility appear to be built into human experience; they provide the framework within which orderly interaction between persons and groups takes place. Such structures seem to be a fundamental requisite for the maintenance of human life in communities. We are at least irked, and at times thrown into chaos, when this fabric of mutual responsibility begins to break down.

It amounts to stating the obvious therefore that the key to effective functioning of human interactions in any given setting is predicated on 'mutual expectation' which when 'habituated,' requires (for the most part) no contract signing or an external force with power of sanction to ensure conformity. This would be the norm except of course when some persons or entities choose to infringe on the rule or standard of behavior shared by members of the social group; in which case, they would be judged untrustworthy and irresponsible. Otherwise put, we constantly face situations in which we must make decisions, hard or simple, on what to do, how, when, etc. And whatever cause of action we choose inevitably carries some repercussions for ourselves, for others around and beyond us, and for the physical environment. In the words of Gustafson and Laney, "Reflection upon responsibility therefore moves between the inward

---

of time. In essence, several aspects of the moral code are based on pan-cultural human psychological characteristics. Also in the same compendium confer, Bierhoff and Auhagen's "Responsibility as a Fundamental Phenomenon;" Birnbacher's "Philosophical Foundations of Responsibility;" and Shaver and Schutte's "Towards a Broader Psychological Foundation for Responsibility: Who, What, How." Shaver and Schutte offer additional explanation as to how the attribution of responsibility provides a broader psychological foundation for the critical aspect of human activity.

5 Merriam-Webster's Collegiate Dictionary. 2005. Eleventh Edition, Massachusetts: Merriam Webster, Inc.

6 Gustafson, James and Laney, James. Eds. 1968. *On Being Responsible: Issues in Personal Ethics*, New York: Harper & Row, Publishers.

look – where we examine ourselves – and the outward survey, where we attempt to appreciate the possibilities open to us within the limits of time and place in which we live."[7]

That responsibility is so fecund is proof that it relentlessly loops with our daily actions (and even inactions). Gustafson and Laney characterize the reflection about different responsibilities as a natural occurrence of daily human experiences. These fleeting human experiences, come in a spectrum, from the 'very unsophisticated' to the 'highly sophisticated and complex' ones; and considerations of weight are judgment calls. For the unsophisticated, we tend to make decisions relatively quickly and on the fly; but sophisticated situations demand (or ought to demand) deeper and more thoughtful deliberations.[8]

Thus far, besides the import that the two authors highlight, namely the centrality of responsibility in the proper functioning of societies, there is the fact that responsibility is more than a *given* of experience. According to them, "it is an *ought* which persons need to be aware of". But I will defer for later discussion the emphasis on the 'ought.'

Being responsible involves a call for a response or a call to action, not merely a reaction. It is that type of responsiveness that is somewhat proactive even as it often comes after the action. Richard Niebuhr and Bernard Haring underscore these interrelated attributes in their respective reflections on responsibility.[9] Christian theological ethicist Niebuhr identifies the symbol of responsibility as containing hidden references, allusions and similes which reside in our minds "as we grope for understanding of ourselves and toward definition of ourselves in action."[10] Similarly, Gustafson and Laney seem to carry the argument further in their claim that, "Fundamental to the notion of action as part of responsibility is the conception of persons who have the capacity (freedom) to govern their responses to what occurs to them, and to give direction to the responses they in turn make."[11]

---

7 Ibid, p. 14.

8 The authors provide sample questions and explanations that serve as guide: "To whom am I responsible? For what am I responsible? By raising these questions, we are forced to make explicit certain things that might have missed our attention. Responsibility is not a *thing*, a substance that is everywhere and always one and the same. It is a relationship between myself and others, or a relationship I have to certain situations." Ibid, p. 7.

9 Niebuhr, Richard. 1968. "The Meaning of Responsibility"; and Haring, Bernard. 1968. "Essential Concepts of Moral Theology." Both in *On Being Responsible: Issues in Personal Ethics*, New York: Harper & Row, Publishers.

10 Niebuhr, p. 20.

11 Ibid, p. 11.

What about other attributes so often associated with responsibility, such as, accountability, obligation, trustworthiness, reliability and fidelity? By associative resonance, the hint is that some of these may ring ancient bells with historical roots to, for instance Aristotle's *Nichomachean Ethics.*[12] In apparent recognition of this Niebuhr aims not to contrive a novel idea but to highlight what has been in existence for centuries and then tie it to real life experiences. At issue are considerations of the process of assessment and interpretation of what is going on in a given moment and the need to respond to situations in light of various commitments and obligations.[13]

Responsible individuals are adjudged to be so because of the faith that is placed on them to live up to a certain level of expected behavior. "They can be expected to keep their commitments and fulfill their obligations unless there is a just cause – a higher obligation – that requires them to violate that trust."[14] An anecdote of a higher obligation looks like this: As a paramount chief, Sagamore Ahiga has campaigned, raised money, and even galvanized his subjects to vote *en masse* for Congressman Ahote. But, to his chagrin, he discovers that Ahote has been propping the interest of the timber industry whose decades-old logging activities have decimated the livelihood of the indigenous people. Normally, the fact that the Sagamore has, for four straight electoral cycles, sustained Ahote's grip on political power with his unflinching support as one of their own, would be a reason to continue in the hope that Ahote will change; but in this situation, it is not. It isn't that the Sagamore and his subjects have *some* reason to return Ahote to office and more reason to put him out. Sagamore Ahiga has no reason at all to return him to office, but instead to build another political alliance that would be answerable,[15] nay, *responsible* to his community's interest and wellbeing.

Hence, this intuition is in consonant with suggestions about responsibility as "obligations that one has by virtue of his commitments, his role in society, his power and authority… Whether one does or does not fulfill these obligations is a point on which we are judged by others and by ourselves."[16]

In discussing "Responsibilities to Persons," Christopher Gowans[17] conceives of a concentric relationship whereby responsibilities to persons tee off from

12 This theme will be explored later.

13 Niebuhr, p. 20.

14 Gustafson and Laney, p. 12.

15 Here, "answerability" or "accountability" can also conjure up such familiar (legal) terms as "liability" "burden" and "obligation." This anecdote was spawned by a similar one by Jonathan Dancy in the book, *Moral Reasons,* Cambridge, Massachusetts: Blackwell, 1993.

16 Ibid. pp. 12–13.

17 Gowans, Christopher. 1994. *Innocence Lost: An Examination of Inescapable Moral Wrongdoing.* New York: Oxford University Press, p. 122.

within one's inner circle and extends to the outer parts – seen also as the proximate to the ultimate, or the nucleus to the periphery paradigm. And as this umbra to the penumbra relationship goes, so does the degree of responsibility fades. He emphasizes the importance of this cognitive framework of responsibility which is initiated with kinship and extends to friendship, social group, citizenship, and so on. This network of relational connections and their concomitant responsibilities are "central to what makes our lives worthwhile, and it is within such relationships that we come to best understand what is involved in the notion of responsibility."[18]

Surely enough, Gowans' paradigm of responsibility resides not just within the individual and his intimates but can (and does) stretch out to a wide array of a network including strangers within the neighborhood or in locales near and far, to the unborn child, to persons in persistent vegetative state, to generations past and future, to non-human animals, to the ecosystem, to a creator, etc. Responsibility in this broader amalgam of chain relationships can as well exist between persons with common interests, needs, beliefs and aspirations. Hence Gowans envisions such umbrella groups as corporations, faith groups, race, ethnicities, professions, social movements, political parties, and schools.[19]

As would be expected these collective groupings differ fundamentally from individual persons in several ways. Thus, Gowans says that, "There is nothing that constitutes a person as persons constitute social entities."[20] This means that, for one, the social entities have overarching objectives that collectively transcend the individual needs of the persons that make them up (such as a community's devotion to a certain time-honored custom). Also, the survival of the social groups is not tied to the membership of some specific persons. This shared fact is one of the key determining factors; that, "our relationships with these groups and responsibilities to them are not reducible to our relationships with and responsibilities to some list of persons."[21] To illustrate, it is totally conceivable that the entire members of a university's Board of Trustees could (God forbid) perish in a plane crash (or abducted by some aliens) with no effect on an ongoing federal investigation into that institution's alleged violations of clinical trial guidelines.

Another relevant tack to Gowans' 'responsibility to persons' framework is his point – a familiar idea in moral philosophy – about the intrinsic value of persons which in other words sees individual persons as valuable in and of themselves. He cleverly avoids the classical epistemological empiricism (with

18 Ibid, p. 129.
19 Ibid, p. 129.
20 Ibid, p. 129.
21 Ibid, p. 130.

reasons such as autonomy, rationality, freedom, and capacity for affection) for this position, thus evading the Myth of the Given; but rationalizes that "it is sufficient to observe that it is a fundamental feature of moral experience that individuals are regarded as valuable in themselves."[22] If this passes for a look-alike notion for Kant's respect for persons as ends in themselves, Gowans is quick to object with a couple of reasons.

One, Kant's metaphysics presupposes a bi-polar world of noumena and phenomena, with only the noumenal person enjoying such attributes as rationality and freedom and by implication is accorded the 'an end-in-itself' status. The 'phenomenal person' (the merely empirical with no moral significance) is excluded. In Gowans' paradigm, the whole person is included along with such things as all the features associated with his particular history and culture.[23] Two, Gowans doesn't endorse Kant's "respect for persons as ends in themselves as a manifestation of respect for the moral law dictated by pure practical reason."[24] Rather, he regards persons as intrinsically valuable not by the application of *a priori* moral law, but through the experience of concrete interaction; in other words, this is determined from particular individual cases. So, while Gowans regards each person as both intrinsically valuable as well as uniquely valuable, for Kant, (*noumenal*) persons are ends in themselves in a way that is unequally shared by all. To nail home the point about the unmatched value of each person, Gowans cites the loss of a mother or a sibling: yes, they could be replaced by a step-mother or a sister, but these are only partial compensations, and he thinks morality must consider this as a central point.[25]

Taken together, on Gowans' account, the potentiality for responsibility is established the instant persons connect through different forms of interactive relationships, and each side should duly be accorded the attributes of being intrinsically and uniquely valuable. This way, persons are beings deserving of certain sense of duty or obligation either through chosen or unchosen circumstance whereby relationships are established, be it via family relationships

---

22 Ibid, p. 123.

23 Ibid, p. 123.

24 Ibid, p. 123.

25 Cognizant that he could be accused of propagating a recipe for prejudice, Gowans labors to make clear that it would be illogical to conclude that the fact that the point is made about the unique value of persons does not make it a tenable argument to regard some persons as more valuable than others; in other words, assigning valency to persons in a stacked order of preference cannot be valid. Thus, he says, "To regard each person as uniquely valuable, and hence as having no relation of comparative value to any person, cannot be a basis for choice." Ibid, p.126.

(proximate) or outside circumstance of common or extended interest (ultimate). I couldn't agree more with this concentric paradigm of responsibility. It could have been hugely problematic if it were restricted only within relations of kinship and friends. Admittedly, and depending on the circumstance, it covers much more – strangers, foreigners, living or dead, unborn or disabled, non-human animals, the environment, and even the spiritual world.

The mission in this book is to re-conceive the concept of responsibility (possibly touching on some of its different forms – legal, moral, etc.). While it is novel particularly given its anchor hook – the role of personhood in African thought – it would be simplistic to assume that there had existed no previous ground breaking philosophical proposals which have sought to re-conceptualize the concept.[26] Emmanuel Levinas' peculiar reversal of the concept is a prime case in point. His unorthodox approach to responsibility has variously been described as an 'about turn,' an 'inversion,' an 'expropriatory' or a 'revolutionary' view. It detaches completely from any in modern Western tradition before him from Descartes to Husserl, in the manner he overturns the superiority of egology and the supremacy of the will.[27] Instead, he posits that responsibility is primordially a being for the other. "No longer a responsibility for oneself or for one's actions, but a responsibility for the other and for the sake of the other; no longer following the freedom of the subject, but arising out of the other's demand on me."[28] It is important to understand that for Levinas, the ethicality of ethics lies in responsibility.[29] And since moral persons are not abstract idealizations but individuals experiencing the physical life, the environment

26 Karin Boxer's (2013) *Rethinking Responsibility,* Oxford University Press, is just but one recent effort at providing a new "perspective on what has become to some a stale dialectic regarding free will and moral responsibility," according to Matt King, UCLA School of Law, a reviewer of that publication.

27 Raffoul, François. 2010. *The Origins of Responsibility,* Indianapolis: Indiana University Press, p. 164. It is noted as well that Levinas' extraordinary thinking on responsibility is patently opposed to Sartre's. "For both, the 'I' carries the weight of the world on its shoulders, but for exactly opposite reasons… whereas Sartre places all the weight on the self and its freedom, Levinas empties such a free subject and expropriates it in favor of the other," p. 165.

28 Ibid, p. 163.

29 Raffoul provides further background about Levinas' mission which was to upend the prevailing philosophical status quo by altering the "traditional hierarchy in which ethics is reduced to being a branch of ontology and epistemology, and seeks to raise ethics to the level of first philosophy." As such, ethics is beyond knowledge, in fact, beyond being. p. 166.

and each other in social systems, responsibility is cardinally significant only if it is to the other; so much so that the most authentic relationship one can have with the other lies in taking upon oneself the fate of the other.[30]

> What makes humans human is the ethical, as responsibility for the other human. Understood in this way, ethics represents what is truly human in human beings, a humanism of the other that breaks with the ego-centered philosophies and opens onto the infinite character of the alterity of the other to whom I am responsible.[31]

In rethinking the totality of ethics and of ethicality itself, and by implication, of responsibility, Levinas' proposal is an explication of responsibility in the context of ethics of hospitality – a pre-originary openness to the other. But quite unlike our normal understanding of a host-guest relationship, Levinas defines the subject as hôte (which in French means both host and guest), that is, the subject is welcome to the other before any self-posited identity or a "pre-given substantial identity that would constitute the basis for a capacity to welcome…; the subject does not pre-exist the encounter with the other but is pre-assigned to the other."[32] This uncanny view of responsibility presents the subject as a host, a guest and a "hostage" – someone who is visited in his home (by a neighbor, a relative, a stranger, an exile, an immigrant) but seems to be in the home of the other and expropriated toward the other for whom he is now obligated.

Levinas' experience of responsibility as a face to face encounter – the irreducible form of relationship – seems to cohere somewhat with the social nature of Gowans' concentric paradigm which starts with the subject's immediate fellow moral agents with whom he/she interacts. Hence, a "face to face" encounter upon which responsibility is rooted is essentially of an ethical nature which is a relation to the other as opposed to some transcendent Good.[33] It is in this meeting that agential emotions are observed, evaluated, exchanged and/or acted upon, be they fragile or virile, vulnerable or secure, as a result of which Levinas calls for the obligation to be responsible for the other.

30 Ibid, pp. 196 and 191.

31 Ibid, p. 168.

32 Ibid, p. 178. Raffoul sees Levinas' definition of the subject as "subject of welcome" much more than just a reversal but an annihilation of Kant's notion of autonomous responsible subject. Confer p. 180.

33 Ibid, p. 184.

In summary, it seems clear that Levinas' radical moral phenomenology borders on the ideal, or even the utopic. But, it is probably something worth aspiring to if we must make progress at prompting a result or achieving a goal. It is the same reason for which movies are exaggerated to jolt the senses and elicit emotional appreciation. Except of course, moral systems are neither staged nor induced to ignite or elicit emotions. This has led authors to canvass that the bars of morality be raised high enough as to lift lousy moral agents from torpor. The view pictures a moral theory in the mold of the Christian religious tradition, for example, the Good Samaritan, or better, Christ's giving up of his life for the salvation of mankind: "Responsibility for the other to the point of dying for the other."[34] If Levinas' precepts were to be realized, human conflicts and suffering would be eternally erased. Otherwise, how do you plot the empirical practicality of a moral system that he envisages? Perhaps, one-word answer would suffice: selflessness. Indeed, the ultimate form of it.

> This responsibility for the other is non-reciprocal, dissymmetrical or asymmetrical, infinite, and non-chosen; it is the experience of a being devoted to the other in the guise of a being "hostage" to the other. All concerns for reciprocity, contracts and agreements with others are inadequate to capture my original responsibility to the other as pre-originary passivity before the infinite obligation to the other...[35]

3.3 Responsibility as a Virtue

To view responsibility within the context of virtue ethics is useful in anchoring my argument and perhaps further crystalize its trajectory. Thus far, whether it be Gowans' espousal of responsibility to fellow moral agents as being intrinsically and uniquely valuable; the obligation to be responsible for the other by Levinas; Gustafson and Laney's exposé of responsibility as an *ought*; or Richard Niebuhr and Bernard Haring's view that responsibility occasions a response or a call to action; all may be judged to exhibit some trappings identifiable with virtue. They all emphasize the acquisition of moral character – an attribute that harks back to Plato and Aristotle (or more accurately with roots in ancient

34 Ibid, p. 196.
35 Ibid, p. 197.

African thought).[36] Not surprisingly, virtue ethics (which has witnessed a rebirth of sorts in recent times[37]) ruminates over such things as,

> …motives and moral character, moral education, moral wisdom or discernment, friendship and family relationships, a deep concept of happiness, the role of the emotions in our moral life and the fundamentally important questions of what sort of person I should be and how we should live… [Virtue] is indeed a character trait, a disposition which is well entrenched in its possessor.[38]

As I have indicated, should we go in search of how responsibility might be rooted in virtue, Aristotle's *Nicomachean Ethics* is *one source* (emphasis intended) that we might resort to.[39] In it, Aristotle espouses to great lengths what virtue is and what it means to be virtuous. Of the two kinds that he identifies, moral virtue (intellectual virtue being the other), is an attribute that is imbibed habitually (etymologically termed *ethiké*, a variant of *ethos*). Moral virtues arise not by nature since nature is a given; instead, nature has adapted humans to receive them, and through habits virtues are made perfect.[40]

36 The *Stanford Encyclopedia of Philosophy* points to ancient Chinese philosophy. Information was accessed at http://plato.stanford.edu/entries/ethics-virtue/ on April 2, 2014. Other more convincing sources point to, believe it or not, ancient African philosophy. For more, see Innocent Onyewuenyi (2005), *The African Origin of Greek Philosophy*, and Cheikh Diop (1974), *The African Origin of Civilization*.

37 Some accounts of this revival can be found in Roger Crisp, "Modern Moral Philosophy and the Virtues." *How Should One Live? Essays on the Virtues*, Crisp, Roger (Ed.), Oxford: Oxford University Press, 1996), 1–18; Gregory Trianosky. 1990. "What is Virtue Ethics All About?" *American Philosophical Quarterly* 27: 335–344; Sosa, E., 1991. *Knowledge in Perspective*. Cambridge: Cambridge University Press; Zagzebski, L. 1996. *Virtues of the Mind*. Oxford: Clarendon Press; Greco, J. 2000. *Putting Skeptics in Their Place*. Cambridge, Cambridge University Press; Greco, J. (Ed.). 2004. *Ernest Sosa and His Critics*. Oxford: Blackwell Publishing; Sosa, E. 2007. *A Virtue Epistemology*. Oxford: Clarendon Press.

38 The online *Stanford Encyclopedia of Philosophy* information was accessed at http://plato.stanford.edu/entries/ethics-virtue/ on April 2, 2014.

39 I have emphasized *one source* for a reason. For starters, the prototype for Aristotle's virtue ethics is the concept of *Maat*, a moral principle that was invented and taught by African priest-philosophers and scientists of the ancient Egyptian Mystery system. Aristotle was a pupil of Plato who in turn learned firsthand, from the Egyptian mystery tradition. Also, Aristotle inherited a massive amount of library and other loots from Alexander the Great after he conquered Egypt in 332 BC. Aristotle was Alexander's home teacher and he (Alexander) greatly admired Aristotle's wits. Get more from *The African Origin of Greek Philosophy* by Innocent Onyewuenyi, 2005, pp. 154–159.

40 *Nichomachean Ethics*, Book II, Section 1.

Virtue according to Aristotle, resides in the states of character and it is by this that we are defined (not by passions – appetite, anger, fear, etc.); nor by faculties – becoming angry or being pained or feeling pity. In other words, being virtuous is both being in a state of character and to what extent we are in that state. Thus, "with reference to anger we stand badly if we feel it violently or too weakly, and well if we feel it moderately."[41] Obviously, this seems to echo the widely-used cliché that virtue is in the middle – mean or intermediate – with 'excess' and 'defect' at both extremes. It can also be viewed that attaining virtue is like aiming at the bull's eye, it is never a goal that is achieved overnight; hence it is by practice (formed over time as a habit) and attained through what Lovibond[42] calls "internalism." In Aristotle's own words,

> That moral virtue is a mean, then, and in what sense it is so, and that it is a mean between two vices, the one involving excess, the other deficiency, and that it is such because its character is to aim at what is intermediate in passions and in actions, has been sufficiently stated. Hence also it is no easy task to be good. For in everything it is no easy task to find the middle, e.g. to find the middle of a circle is not for everyone but for him who knows; so, too, anyone can get angry- that is easy- or give or spend money; but to do this to the right person, to the right extent, at the right time, with the right motive, and in the right way, that is not for everyone, nor is it easy; wherefore goodness is both rare and laudable and noble.[43]

Thus, in exact same way, appropriate sense of responsibility, for instance, would be cultivated and habituated over time. And it makes a difference if fostered early on in one's youth or developmental training regardless of one's professional calling.

On this much, morality is firmly rooted in human nature such that to live a good and rewarding life entails living in accordance with virtue. However, that goodness of character, is formed by learned customary practice or behavioral response.[44]

Still, there is more to be said about Aristotle's two-part domains of virtue.

> Virtue… consists of two kinds, intellectual virtue and moral virtue. Intellectual virtue or excellence owes its origin and development chiefly to teaching, and for that reason requires experience and time. Moral

41 Ibid: Section 5.

42 For a detailed overview see Sabina Lovibond's *Ethical Formation,* 2002.

43 Aristotle's *Nichomachean Ethics*, Section 9.

44 Cahn, S. 2008. *Seven Masterpieces of Philosophy*. New York: Pearson Longman, p. 34.

> virtue, on the other hand, is formed by habit, *ethos*, and its name, *ēthike'*, is therefore derived by a slight variation, from *ethos*. This shows, too, that none of the moral virtues is implanted in us by nature.[45]

In apparent adoption of this view, Lovibond explains that the "Aristotelian ancestry of the concept of (moral) virtue traditionally consists – under one aspect – in a capacity for *thinking correctly* about how to respond to particular situations as they arise. (This is the capacity summed up in the concept of *phronēsis,* a 'practical wisdom' – in Aristotle's term, an 'intellectual,' not a 'moral' virtue, but one that has to be understood by abstracting the common cognitive element from a range of different virtues that are genuinely moral: virtues consisting in the reliable disposition to deal in an appropriate, felicitous, or at least not contemptible way with the various sorts of circumstances attendant on human life)."[46]

Virtue ethics, then, can be seen as aiming at the evaluation of the rational character ideal as it relates to practical rationality, and within practical rationality, to the proper appreciation of those (potentially action-guiding) values that lie beyond the range of ordinary self-interest. In formulating this thesis, Lovibond relies in some good measure on other philosophical icons such as David Hume, along with Emmanuel Kant, John McDowell; Alasdair MacIntyre; Martha Nussbaum; and, David Wiggins.[47]

From all indications, this is an effort to revive and rebrand the Platonic-Aristotelian ethical tradition and rejuvenate the account that forms its arrowhead, specifically, that moral virtue is the outcome of a successful process of formation. Hence, "virtue ethics…offers a character ideal not just in the edifying sense (an example we should strive to imitate) but also in an epistemological one: it follows Aristotle in holding out a standard of correct judgment."[48]

Properly considered, the ancient notion of virtue ethics ought to be connected with what it is today as Philip Cafaro[49] has done:

> Most modern ethical theories have been deontological in both form and content. Aristotle's central question is: What is the good life for a human being? Kant and Mill's central question is: What are our duties to

45 Ibid, p. 51.

46 Lovibond, pp. 10–11.

47 Ibid, p. 12.

48 Ibid, p. 14.

49 Cafaro, Philip. 1997. "Virtue Ethics (Not Too) Simplified." *Auslegung: A Journal of Philosophy,* 22: 49–67.

> our fellow human being... The most important consequence of the turn towards virtue ethics [or its resurgence] has been to reopen Aristotle's question... In reasserting the importance of the realm of judgments concerning our flourishing, excellence, and happiness, virtue ethics reclaims for us this neglected half of our ethical lives for intelligent, philosophical consideration.

Enough has already been said to make it clear, I hope, that virtue ethics presents some sort of an outline demanding of continuous moral growth as well as a disposition expressed as an ideal and an achievement. "Cultivating a virtuous disposition entails habituating our emotions in particular ways as well as the exercise of practical reasoning (deliberative judgment, *phronēsis*) so as to learn how and why to act the right way in any given situation, as well as, more broadly, conduct our lives in such a way as to reveal our dedication to (the fundamental value of) the Good."[50] To assist in realizing this supposed target, there is the presupposition that virtue ethics is beholden to the presence of virtuous agents as intimate role models in the form of family members, teachers, peers, etc., who contribute to a person's character formation (formally and informally).[51]

To fashion a fitting alignment between responsibility and virtue, a recourse to a couple of responsibility's close cousins such as reliability and trust, might help. Just like reliability, the concept of responsibility is both central in contemporary moral systems and important for the moral assessment of persons and certain entities (perhaps much more so in some instances). Robert Audi's[52] rendering of reliable persons as people we can count on, is something that would not be possible without the inculcation of virtue and realized through reasoned assessment and voluntary choices. Likewise, we can speak of counting on a reliable person in the same way as we can speak of trusting them. "Counting on people is a way of trusting them... We usually speak of such people only in relation to moral appraisal. The virtue – and the duties – of fidelity are the chief normative notions pertinent to understanding trustworthiness in persons."[53] How someone chooses to follow through or not keep faith with

50 "Virtue Ethics: An Introduction – Part 1," *Ratio Juris: Law, Politics, Philosophy,* October 09, 2009. http://ratiojuris.blogspot.com/2009/10/virtue-ethics-introductionpart-1.html. Viewed on April 09, 2014.

51 Ibid.

52 Audi, Robert. 2009. "Reliability as a Virtue." *Philosophical Studies*, 142: 43.

53 Ibid, p. 52.

commitments and responsibilities usually weighs heavily toward their character vis-a-vis the sorts of commitments and responsibilities he/she takes.[54]

Virtuous acts don't occur by happenstance, they are willed and exercised by the agent's judgment. Therefore, if living a virtuous life typifies our innate excellences (aretaié, areté) which hankers for the Good, and responsibility is essentially other-regarding and through which we are fulfilled, then the basis for responsibility as a virtue is thus established. Just like Levinas, Julia Annas is of the view that "in an ethics of virtue there is no room for supererogation".[55] In this way one of the major criticisms leveled against virtue ethics (of being self-centered) is voided. For as Nafsika Athanasoulis, a moral theorist and applied philosopher says, demands of morality and a moral agents' individual interests do not conflict. While the good life for humans is the life of virtue, it is as well in our interest to be virtuous.

> The virtues are other-regarding. Kindness, for example, is about how we respond to the needs of others. The virtuous agent's concern is with developing the right sort of character that will respond to the needs of others in an appropriate way. The virtue of kindness is about being able to perceive situations where one is required to be kind, have the disposition to respond kindly in a reliable and stable manner, and be able to express one's kind character in accordance with one's kind desires. The eudaemonist account of virtue ethics claims that the good of the agent and the good of others are not two separate aims. Both rather result from the exercise of virtue. Rather than being too self-centered, virtue ethics unifies what is required by morality and what is required by self-interest.[56]

In a nutshell, virtue ethics essentially aims to examine and determine the character ideal in relation to practical rationality, "to the proper appreciation of those (potentially action-guiding) values that lie beyond the range of ordinary self-interest."[57]

54 Kupperman, Joel. 1991. *Character*. New York: Oxford University Press.

55 Annas, Julia. 1993. *The Morality of Happiness*. New York: Oxford University Press.

56 See Nafsika Athanasoulis' contribution in the *Internet Encyclopedia of Philosophy*: A Peer-reviewed Academic resource. Accessed at http://www.iep.utm.edu/virtue/ on April 09, 2014.

57 Lovibond, p. 11.

3.4 Corporate Responsibility

In the preceding sections, I have tried to articulate albeit cursorily, given the magnitude of the literary corpus, the concept of responsibility mostly at the individual level. In this concluding part of the chapter I will try to summatively consider responsibility at the corporate level. Here, references to the term 'corporate' loosely refers to any form of grouping of persons such as in corporations and organizations, commercial firms, political parties, nation states, government departments, religious groups, trade unions and similar assemblages or aggregations. As such these are legal entities and group agents. Also, the discussion is with a hindsight on the ascription of corporations as legal persons or legal entities.[58]

Right off the bat, I acknowledge that this can pose an extremely knotty discussion, particularly when social responsibility is considered alongside with roles of corporations. Questions that crop up are quotidian. They include, are corporations persons (do they exhibit capacities associated with personhood)? Should corporations have morality; or do they belong to the moral community? Should corporations be held socially responsible? These recurrent questions might be trite but they are unavoidable and touch on the core of the main case study of this work. I have in mind the hugely controversial clinical trial protocol by the multinational drug maker Pfizer, in Nigeria in 1996, (details in Chapter 1). On the broad-based universally accepted standards that group agents should be held responsible for their actions, this book argues that the apparent brazen conduct of that clinical protocol in 1996 – administration of the experimental drug Trovan, to a large number of pediatric patients – provides yet another powerful reason to revisit the concept of corporate responsibility in an attempt to reconceptualize and redefine it.

Also, it should be borne in mind that synonymous to corporate responsibility is the concept of collective (legal, moral, social) responsibility. Presently,

58 French, Peter. 1991. "The Corporation as a Moral Person." *Collective Responsibility: Five Decades of Debate in Theoretical and Applied Ethics*, Larry May and Stacey Hoffman, (Eds.), p. 133. Suffice it to add that French's position has for over 30 years, metamorphosed from referring to corporations as "moral persons," to calling them "moral actors." For more see the analysis "Collective Moral Responsibility" by David Risser, 2009. When he did, French, a towering figure in the collective responsibility debate assigned legal personhood to corporations on the basis that corporations are "members of the moral community, of equal standing with the traditionally acknowledged residents: biological human beings. He traces its origin to the Roman, through the English legal systems, and to what is today widely understood by a juristic person as "any entity that is a subject of right"; p. 136.

I aim to pitch in my 'two cents' to the poser about whether or not corporations have other responsibilities (for instance, social responsibility) in addition to the responsibility to generate revenue for their owners and shareholders.

In the introduction to this chapter, I might have blown the tops on whose side I'm on in this debate by stating my point-blank opposition to the argument that shields corporations from social responsibility merely on the claim that profit-making trumps everything else. But I'm pretty comfortable doing so right at the outset. I can't keep my intuition from rationalizing in any other way: corporations, large and small, public and private, ought to make provision to embed social responsibility (among other responsibilities) in their operational policies and practices. In fact, as a matter of common sense, to do otherwise in this day and age, namely, sole pursuit of maximum profits and expansion of shareholder base, would be injudicious.

For a rehash, the claim that maximizing profits is the same thing as being socially responsible probably originates from Adam Smith's "laissez-faire economic" argument. In it, Smith posits that businesses are in and of themselves socially responsible just by pursuing their own self-interest. This is why businesses are easily touted as job boosters and economic developers locally, regionally and globally.

After contesting this Smithian position, James Roper[59] considers the question whether it is even possible for a corporation to be socially responsible without jeopardizing its own existence – or worse. He examines several arguments to this conclusion, but I will mention just a few. One, a corporation that engages in ethically beneficial acts that reduce profits will be vulnerable to stiff resistance by shareholders. Roper cites the early 20th Century suit by the Dodge brothers (who owned stocks in Ford Motor Company) against Henry Ford's plan to build housing for his auto workers. When matters could not be settled in the lower courts, the U.S. Supreme Court decided against Ford on the grounds that his action would reduce shareholder dividends. In hindsight, that decision was ill-informed.

Two, a corporation that engages in ethically beneficial acts that reduced profits will be vulnerable to a hostile takeover by another competition with the intent of breaking it up and dismantling any ethically desirable structures the corporation might have instituted. The obvious fallacy in this argument is that of *non-sequitur*. Why must it be assumed that whenever a corporation engages in ethically beneficial acts, it must necessarily lead to reduced profits?

59 Roper, James. 2012. *The Covenant of Democracy: Should Government by Run Like a Business?*" US: Kendall Hunt Publishing Company.

It seems to put beyond our imagination, the possibility of any other option being the case. Wrong.

Three, from the stand point of "market failures," it is argued that public goods cannot come from corporations (at least not at socially optimal levels), because corporations are 'inherently incapable' of being socially responsible. 'Socially optimal level' is a delineation with a utilitarian underpinning but which in turn stems from the kinds of deontological considerations that play a profound role in the U.S. Constitution. Economists refer to "social optimality" in utilitarian terms, but Roper's use of the term refers to deontological considerations that play a profound role in the Constitution of the U.S. Also, the 'inherent incapacitation' here is meant to show that the duty of providing social responsibility is inconsistent with the traditional roles of corporations. In other words, that provision of social responsibility belongs as part of government services, as in the mold of providing for public health, security, and education.

Roper may be right that Smith's arguments regarding social responsibility are flawed, but I contest his own (Roper's) claim that it is not possible for a corporation to be socially responsible. In rejecting Smith, he goes too far in the other direction. I will show in what follows that it is not only possible, it is even desirable for a corporation to be socially responsible in the sense of acting ethically – not in the Smithian sense of simply maximizing profits. Roper and others would probably reply that the ethical actions of a major corporation may simply be part of their marketing strategy since being perceived to be unethical is terrible for business. I am not cynical as to view corporate acts through such a jaded lens.

The vehemence with which these and other arguments have been pushed in favor of profit making ensures that the heat from the collective responsibility debate is unlikely to simmer soon. But, the infixed tussle continually calls for appropriate arrangements in response to some of the effects of the actions of corporations. While some of the actions associated with corporations and other organized collective groups are quite beneficial, others have certainly constituted widespread harm and wrongdoing. In his reflection, David Risser[60] aims to provide a platform on which to explain the bone of contention between methodological individualists for whom all social phenomena are explained by reference to individual moral agents; and methodological holists

60 Risser, David. "Collective Moral Responsibility" on the Internet Encyclopedia of Philosophy. Accessed at http://www.iep.utm.edu/virtue/ on April 09, 2014.

who contend that actions by social groups “cannot be reduced to the actions and interests of their individual members.”[61]

> Collective moral responsibility raises disagreement between conceptions of collective responsibility which maintain that only individual human agents can be held morally responsible, and conceptions which maintain that groups, such as corporations, can be held morally responsible as groups, independently of their members.[62]

Risser relies on Joel Feinberg’s[63] taxonomy of collective responsibility to execute this task. There, Feinberg posits a set of four arrangements beginning with “Group Liability without Fault” in which the entire group is held morally responsible for the actions of either a single member, a coterie few, or the whole members. Just by its very nature, namely of subsuming the individual autonomy within the group, Risser is of the opinion that this arrangement seems to collide with Western individualism and bodes well with more communitarian societies such as found in parts of Africa and Asia. But it is important to position this type of arrangement within groups that show appreciable level of community of purpose and bonded by common interest such that both benefits and harms are collectively shared.

I find Risser’s illustration of this type of arrangement with Africa and Asia a bit off-color as it seems to exhibit veiled racism and banal understanding of these societies. Otherwise, one wonders why he thinks this could only fit with such “tribes… where conditions are frequently so harsh and barren that life depends on groups sticking together, it is accepted practice for a family, a clan, or a tribe to be held liable and to be punished for the wrongdoing of one of its members.” Miffed, one is bound to ask: why would rational human agents first have to experience harsh life conditions before they see the need for solidarity among their members? And why would this be found only in African and Asian societies? Interestingly, even as Risser has identified the practice of collective responsibility in some Western organizations, e.g., the U.S. military, he nevertheless insists that this arrangement is clearly unsuitable for *most human communities* (my emphasis); oblivious that Africa and Asia constitute overwhelming majority of mankind. He is way off the beam with that argument.

61 Ibid.

62 Ibid.

63 Feinberg, Joel. 1970. “Collective Responsibility.” *Doing and Deserving: Essays in the Theory of Responsibility*. Princeton: Princeton University Press, pp. 222–251.

Feinberg's second arrangement, "Group Liability with Contributory and Non-contributory Fault" refers to some sort of common vices – say, binge drinking, recreational drug peddling, and over speeding – which though frequently committed by the citizenry, are however not always punished. With the example of driving under the influence, Feinberg quips that, "Most of us are 'guilty' of this practice, although only the motorist actually involved in the accident is guilty of the resultant injury. He is guilty ... and more harm is his fault, but it does not necessarily follow that he is guiltier or more at fault than the rest of us."[64] And this can as well be said of what happens with researchers who flout clinical trial protocols. As made clear in Chapter 1; despite the established guidelines for the protection of patient-subjects in research, breaches of certain aspects of research protocols still occur. The main difference between a drunken driver and an errant researcher is that one is impaired by alcohol, the other is though inspired but 'impaired' by rampant desire for fame and profits.

"Group Liability with the Contributory of Every Member," Feinberg's third arrangement, is a composite that corrals together all manner of loose collectives from mob formations, to improvised or fleeting teams or clubs. A group of soccer or basketball enthusiasts who regularly gather to play at a certain time and place (say, on Saturday mornings at a public park) might serve as a good example. It is conceivable that such a group can gang up to harm or discriminate against someone on gender or racial grounds. The relevant question that Risser raises is how moral responsibility could be shared among members of a random aggregate such as this. Just like Feinberg, Virginia Held and Larry May have weighed in in search of answers but they all struggle with the thorny issue of adequately assigning moral responsibility to individual members in a group. Feinberg,[65] and to some extent May[66] seem to agree that the group ring leaders ought to bear greater responsibility than passive participants who might have simply tagged along in the act. Risser summates and I agree that, "Degree judgments of blame present even greater challenges because they are based on each member's intentions and state of mind... [Nonetheless] this factor must always be included in moral responsibility judgments and may mitigate or aggregate an agent's responsibility and blameworthiness."[67]

64 Ibid, p. 242.

65 Feinberg, Joel. 1970. "Collective Responsibility." *Doing and Deserving: Essays in the Theory of Responsibility*. Princeton: Princeton University Press, pp. 222–251.

66 May, Larry. 1992. *Sharing Responsibility*. Chicago: University of Chicago Press.

67 Risser, David. "Collective Moral Responsibility," on the Internet Encyclopedia of Philosophy. Accessed at http://www.iep.utm.edu/virtue/ on April 09, 2014.

Both Held[68] and Michael Zimmerman[69] are of the view that moral responsibility should be shared equally among actors in a wrongdoing. But, on the issue of appropriate distribution of moral responsibility, Held, thinks that the mere presence of any member actor while the group developed and/or carried out a method of action is enough for judging culpability in the group action.

Lastly, Feinberg's forth proposal, "Group Liability with Collective, Non-distributive Fault" presents a collective responsibility arrangement that shields ascription of culpability for an individual or members of a group for a bad action. The fact that government obligation to provide certain services is a continuous irreducible function irrespective of who is in authority at any given time could be a fitting illustration; just as it is the responsibility of the Board of Directors of a company to carry through a decided course of actionable policy by its previous members. Or to use Feinberg's example of a philosophy department that fails to keep faith with its policy of finding substitute faculty personnel to assist with a student's dissertation after two of his committee members had left the department. In any of those cases, organizations ought to keep their commitments regardless of a change of guards. This is a view that resonates or finds expression in Gowans' point that the survival or continued activities of a given social group is not validated or tied to the membership of some specific persons. In other words, there is a moral obligation for continuity of purpose in establishments. Also, no member or members should be indispensable.

I return to briefly address the three niggling questions posed earlier: 1. Are group agents or corporations, persons (do they exhibit capacities associated with personhood)? Let's consider an example: when we say that 'the U.S. Securities and Exchange Commission has *accused* Citigroup of *lying* to investors in a 2007 deal where it *sold* subprime mortgages that it *knew* would default;' is it not obvious that both SEC and Citigroup do exhibit capacities (in asterisks) attributable to personhood?

This was part of the tasks Christian List and Philip Pettit set for themselves as they probed the historicity of the problem of responsibility. In the book, *Group Agency*, the authors hold that the classical connection between corporate responsibility and personhood has roots in 1246 when Pope Innocent IV referred to group agents as fictional or artificial persons without souls. But while disagreeing that they are fictional, List and Pettit concede that corporations are artificial persons, and that it is in that capacity that they can be

68 Held, Virginia. 1970. "Can a Random Collective be Morally Responsible?" *Journal of Philosophy*, 67: 471–481.

69 Zimmerman, Michael. 1985. "Sharing Responsibility." *American Philosophical Quarterly*, 22: 115–122.

considered as institutional or juristic persons.[70] The authors adopt this position, which I endorse, based not on the intrinsic nature or character of corporations, but by what they do extrinsically, the roles they play or the functions they discharge; hence, it is the performative conception. This legal approach (later adopted as a philosophical thought), which derived from the Roman law during the Middle Ages, sees the legal person as follows:

> An entity capable of legal rights and duties: an entity that can own, buy and sell, enter into contracts and sue for breach of contract, or otherwise have standing as a plaintiff or defendant in the courts. This legal sense of personhood focuses on what persons do rather than what they are. It allows that an entity may be a legal person without being a natural person like an individual human being. To be a person on this conception, does not depend on the stuff out of which one is made but only on one's performance, specifically one's performance in the space of social norms.[71]

There is little wonder therefore why contemporary legal provisions allow corporations to perform many of the things attributable to human persons and regularly accord them the status of 'persons.'[72] Instances where corporations are protected in the U.S. legal system include the 14th amendment to the Constitution. That amendment which came on the heels of the Civil War, gave the freed slaves the standing and protection of other natural persons. And from 1886, when the Supreme Court decided in the *Santa Clara County vs. Southern Pacific Railroad*, "it was taken by the courts to give a comparable standing to corporations."[73]

More recently, some have argued that corporations can even "vote" by other means; something that was inconceivable not too long ago. They invoke for instance, the affirmation in 2010 by the U.S. Supreme Court of the right of

---

70 List, Christian, and Pettit, Philip. 2011. *Group Agency: The Possibility, Design, and Status of Corporate Agents*. Oxford: Oxford University Press, p. 155. The widening spread of the legal origins of the edification of the corporations got a boost back in 1444 in the provisions of the Rolls of British Parliament from where it evolved further spreading to France, Germany and the rest of the world. Read more in Sanford Schane's 1986 article, "The Corporation is a Person."

71 Ibid, pp. 171–172.

72 Hager, M. 1989. "Bodies Politic: The Progressive History of Organizational 'Real Entity' Theory." *University of Pittsburg Law Review*. 50:575–654.

73 Ibid, p. 175. Get additional detail at *Justia US Supreme Court*: Santa Clara County vs. Southern Pacific R. Co., 118 U.S. 394 (1886). Viewed on August 29, 2014 at, https://supreme.justia.com/cases/federal/us/118/394/case.html.

corporations to express their political views in the unrestricted campaign contributions they make to political parties (in the *Citizens United vs.* FEC case).

Other analysts indicate to the contrary that this claim seems a bit stretched. Nonetheless, what is undebatable is the impact political war chest can sometimes have on election outcomes. Perhaps a far more exerting anthropomorphization of corporations is the June 2014 decision of the U.S. apex court in the case of *Burwell vs. Hobby Lobby, Inc.* The Supreme Court ruled 5–4, that requiring family-owned corporations to pay for insurance coverage for contraception under the Affordable Care Act violated a federal law protecting religious freedom. In essence, the court ruled that some corporations (for instance, the ones that are owned or controlled by religious groups or families) have religious beliefs, just like ordinary flesh and blood persons. Such corporations cannot be required to provide contraceptive coverage for their female employees against the beliefs of their owners. At issue are regulations promulgated by the Department of Health and Human Services under the Patient Protection and Affordable Care Act of 2010, which requires specified employers' group health plans to furnish preventive care and screenings for women without any cost sharing requirements.

Opponents contend that this decision violates Religious Freedom Restoration Act, of 1993 which prohibits the "Government [from] substantially burden[ing] a person's exercise of religion even if the burden results from a rule of general applicability..."

> The *Citizens United vs.* FEC case is quite telling.
>
> If group agents can do this, then they have to count as persons, albeit ones of an institutional rather than a biological kind... with basic pre-requisites of personhood. Not only do they form and enact a single mind... displaying beliefs and desires and acting on their basis. They can speak for that mind in a way that enables them to function within the space of mutually recognized obligations.[74]

It needs explicating further that having basic pre-requisites of personhood does not put group agents in exact same status as normal persons with flesh and blood. They are pachydermic and rigid in a number of ways, and lack the perceptive and emotive attributes of human individuals.[75] Such rights and privileges that are not obliged to corporations include, the ability to marry or

74 List and Pettit, pp. 176–177.

75 Ibid, p. 176.

be married, adopt children, be voted for or run a government, and the right to education. But despite the abundance of dissimilarities between a corporation and a flesh-and-blood human, there are enough resembling attributes that have made the law to regard the corporation as a person,[76] thus making it a vastly well accepted artificial, but not fictional person. So, without a doubt, I affirm that corporations are persons, but they are persons in the performative sense that I have espoused.

2. Should corporations be held responsible (legally, morally, socially, etc.)? Put in another way, can group agents be subjected to disciplinary treatment and deprived, restricted or punished as a result of some irresponsible conduct? This is a question that requires extensive deliberation. But, I'd rather cut to the chase. Legally: the short answer is yes, history is dotted with innumerable instances. For instance, in August 2014, Bank of America agreed to pay almost $17 billion in a settlement with the U.S. Justice Department, much of which was used for consumer relief for the bank's mistreatment of its mortgage lenders. Morally: I'd answer yes as well, and my rationale is lumped with the answer to the third question below. Socially: certainly yes, corporations ought to be socially responsible particularly given their power and influence in contemporary business environment. Unlike the early 19th century era when legislative acts allowed the establishment of corporations only within closely defined terms; the gradual relaxation of regulations which led to the explosion of commercial corporations in the latter half of the century and onwards to the 20th and 21st centuries changed all that.[77] That development proved to be the precursor, a harbinger of sorts, to the present day globalization of free market economy – the somewhat idealized transactional or economic regime based on supply and demand with little or no government control. It is the unbridled economic climate where anyone can freely buy, sell, or trade sometimes with little or no state intervention in the form of taxes, subsidies or regulation. This has occasioned a groundswell of an atmosphere of survival of the fittest where powerful corporations easily suck up weaker ones and metamorphose into multinational behemoths with unimaginable power and clout. To put it in perspective,

> Think of the small country where the corporation would trigger an enormous crisis by moving elsewhere, as it is always free to do. Or think of the community that has suffered serious or other environmental harm

76 Schane, Sanford. 1986. "The Corporation is a Person: The Language of a Legal Fiction." *Tulane Law Review*, 61, p. 563.

77 Ibid, p. 184.

> at the hands of a corporation, and even if it is successful in the courts, finds itself thwarted by endless appeals and other legally rigged delays in payment. Or think of those in government who depend on the financial support of corporations in their electoral campaigns and dare not get a corporation offside.[78]

In defense of corporate power, some have argued that the fact of possessing power does not imply that that power is always used or misused. To refute that, I would point out that even when this power is not applied it is ever present and continues to radiate disabling fear in individuals, communities and other entities. Operating as silently as gravity, List and Pettit describe it as "power at its most perfect: power that does not need to be actively exercised to have an effect."[79] That much power (and any power, for that matter) cannot afford to be wielded without some responsibility. Plus, we must not be fooled to think that self-restraint is enough to constrain excessive power; after all, if you are a hammer, everything tends to look like a nail.

3. Do, or should corporations have morality (and is the morality of the constituent elements in a corporation equivalent or reducible to the group agents)? My immediate response is to use the cliché: if it walks like a duck and quacks like a duck, then it must be a duck. However, I would insert a proviso: just like in the first question above, group agents are deemed as having morals in the actions they exhibit or the functions they discharge (hence, in the performative sense). My proposition can be expressed in the following simple syllogism:

A. If corporations or group agents (as legal persons) can be held responsible and punished under the law.
B. And, laws are often evaluated on moral grounds or by morality (descriptively or normatively)
C. Then, corporations or group agents have morality.

I can clearly see how my reasoning would conflict with John Ladd's[80] who characterizes corporations as "directed organizations" (a term adopted by James Roper[81]) with maximum profit making as the primary pursuit of their operations.

78 Ibid, p. 184.

79 Ibid, p. 184.

80 Ladd, John. 1970. "Morality and the Ideal of Rationality in Formal Organizations." *The Monist*, 54, 4:488–516.

81 Roper, James. 2012. *The Covenant of Democracy: Should Government by Run Like a Business?"* US: Kendall Hunt Publishing Company.

He claims that ancillary goals such as the growing of their market share, are mere appendages to this primary goal. "It follows that the things these companies do are *hypothetically* related to their goal of maximizing profits. Therefore, these ... businesses are not part of our moral community."[82] Not so fast.

Let's keep in mind that morality refers to a set of codes which govern agential conducts in terms of whether they are good or bad. In exercising such characteristics attributable to human persons, group agents or corporations can create or shed jobs; establish scholarships/trust funds, fellowships; apply aggressive strategies that defraud or reward clients; pollute or clean the environment; engage in or discourage racist or sexist policies that discriminate (or accommodate); institute policies that favor the elite or policies that encourage minorities, etc. These are moral conducts and are clearly performative activities that take place daily in the space of social norms. In fact, rather than become "responsibility defusing machines," as Roper[83] has stated given the way corporate law has evolved, I contend that group agents as legal entities should be assuming more responsibilities, not less. As I have argued above, these responsibilities cover such spheres as legal, social and moral. And indeed, given the broadening interpretation and the permutation of the law over time, the "moral corporation" that Roper suggests has already witnessed a reinvention of sorts to the extent that much of the corporate law doesn't need to be "radically changed in order for corporations to operate in a more ethics friendly environment."[84]

The journalist and author of *The Impulse Society*,[85] Paul Roberts, has spoken up about something many are hesitant to acknowledge: that the pursuit of short-term self-gratification, something that was once scorned as a sign of personal weakness, has now become the default principle for all sectors of our society. This is showing up in individuals, in our financial markets, and in institutions that we have traditionally relied on to curb impulsiveness.

On Roberts' account, this trend went into the overdrive in the latter part of the 20th century with the industrial revolution, the computer revolution, the financial revolution, etc., whereby profits (for example, quarterly financial earnings) and share price became the dominant factors of consideration while all other considerations are put aside. And what is radical about this is that for most of the earlier part of the century, most corporations were the stewards of long-term thinking. They made long-term investments on factories,

82 Ibid: 70.

83 Ibid: 77.

84 Ibid: 82.

85 Roberts, Paul. 2014. *The Impulse Society: America in the Age of Instant Gratification*, New York, NY: Bloomsbury.

innovations, employee training, etc. And almost overnight, all that is thrown out because they now must focus almost entirely on the next quarter's earnings, and a lot of that is attained not with good social impacts.[86]

In light of positioning corporate entities as legal persons, I readily adopt Risser's outlining of the three criteria that organizations should have in order to be considered as morally responsible: (1) Corporations must be intentional agents able to act. (2) They must be able to conform to rules and appreciate the effects of their actions on other individuals, groups and the environment. (3) They must be capable of responding to moral censure with corrective measures.[87] While these conditions seem like a fair prescription, the "status of formal organizations and specifically corporations, has remained at center stage, and the question of whether some organizations can be morally responsible is seen to hinge on questions of the metaphysical identity of organizations."[88]

But in a dog-eat-dog world where persons (individual or corporate) do whatever it takes to get ahead, contending views on this matter are certain to continue particularly from opponents of corporate responsibility. For instance, Eric Palmer[89] once stated starkly that both Michael Jensen and Milton Friedman – two of the most prominent objectors of corporate moral responsibility – think that it is irresponsible for corporations to be socially or morally responsible. Their familiar but dubious reasons include, considerations for high importance of freedoms, and preservation of shareholder value.[90] As noted, they overlook significant possibilities that undermine their fundamental values. This may be unsettling and downright subversive of the long-term common good.

---

86 Most of this narrative derive from my verbatim notes during the PBS broadcast. More details can be obtained online at *Well Read*, http://www.tvw.org/index.php?option=com_tvwplayer&eventID=2015020019. Accessed on February 5, 2015.

87 Risser, David. "Collective Moral Responsibility" on the *Internet Encyclopedia of Philosophy*. Accessed at http://www.iep.utm.edu/virtue/ on April 09, 2014.

88 Ibid.

89 Palmer, Eric. 2010. "Corporate Responsibility and Freedom: A New Argument." 7th IDEA International Conference proceedings in ethics and international development on accountability, responsibility, and integrity in development: The Ethical Challenges in Sub-Saharan Africa and beyond: From 19th-22nd July 2006, Rukooko, Byaruhanga (Ed.), Makerere University, Kampala, Uganda.

90 Ibid, p. 140. And as James White reveals in his *Contemporary Moral Problems*, 1988: 180, opponents of the "doctrine of social responsibility" are equally averse to suggestions which include such things as the duty to reduce [environmental] pollution or elimination of racial and sexual discrimination at work places, all in a bid to prop up profits.

Let me make one more point by way of a question: Does ethics pay? Certainly, when so much weight is attached to immediate profits there is a danger to lose sight of the greater benefits of planning for the long run. "Economists refer to the long run as the time it takes fixed costs to become immediately variable. Though it is usually much shorter and, on rare occasions slightly longer, the long run is generally about seven years... In the long run [corporate social responsibility] will actually raise the company's profits and justify its actions."[91] Roper's claim here is an empirical one and I disagree with it. To reiterate, CSR ought to be seen as short-term pain for long-term gain. As I see it, the sooner entrepreneurships started infusing from the ground up, ethical virtues with economic principles, the better they would realize what a win-win vantage position they assume.

Stephen Hicks speaks likewise in his recommendation for more of business ethics; noting that business ethics' core application purposes are to stop predatory practices and, encourage philanthropy and charity by business.[92] Doing so would entrench more of ethical behavior including the basic mission of business.[93] This is crucial because what is apparent in the argument for the rejection of CSR, is the presumed fear that moral considerations would detract from the primary aim of doing business which is to make profits. Whereas, under a careful scrutiny, it is clear that the mission of ethics is not antithetical to applied disciplines like business in capitalistic societies. In fact, the two are not at cross purposes; they are complementary and mutually beneficial to each other.

It is almost farcical that while some ardent theorists are busy defending the indefensible, many corporations have wisely moved on. Many of those corporate entities now have dedicated policies that front such things as rich cultural exchange within the communities where they operate to ensure that positive benefits transpire; promotion of long-term sustainability and stewardship; adequate engagement with stakeholders, including employees; and, sustainable commitment to curb environmental impact. As guest of Fairmont Hotel in Chicago, I was thrilled to read this on the hotel's brochure.[94]

Come to think of it, there is hardly any way around conducting business today and staying afloat to harvest profits tomorrow without some appreciable

91 James Roper, 2013.

92 Hicks, Stephen. 2009. "What Business Ethics Can Learn from Entrepreneurship." *The Journal of Private Enterprise* 24(2), 2009, p. 49.

93 Robin, D. 2009. "Toward an Applied Meaning for Ethics in Business." *Journal of Business Ethics*, 89:139.

94 See more at http://www.fairmont.com/corporate-responsibility/responsible-business/ Viewed on July 9, 2015.

infusion and adherence to ethical standards and social responsibility. It takes nothing to see that doing otherwise can only mean exhibiting lack of foresight. It takes only but one error or the flouting of the law such as negligence or lax adherence to regulations,[95] for the errant organization to turn around and make painful compensations, beat back bad publicity, strive to burnish and recover public image, before they can start making profits again. Here are two illustrative examples: The 2010 BP oil spill on the U.S. Gulf of Mexico. As I write, BP is reeling under the weight of that crass negligence of drilling regulations. It is the biggest accidental oil spill the world has ever seen which began with the explosion of the Deepwater Horizon in which 11 crew members were killed. The gusher flowed for 87 days and thousands of businesses suffered along an oily arc from Texas to Florida. The resulting environmental impact is still hard to gauge. So big is the ongoing compensation that the oil giant has agreed to pay the largest settlement in U.S. history – $54 billion (and counting).

Also, in January 2015, the Nigerian arm of the Anglo-Dutch energy giant Royal Dutch Shell agreed to pay, following a six-year legal battle, the record-setting amount of about $84 million to Bodo, a Nigerian fishing community devastated by two serious oil spills in 2008. The compensation will go to 15,600 Nigerian fishermen and farmers whose livelihoods were affected and to the wider community.[96]

Why the fuss you might ask; and why do we have to prove an axiom in defense against the onslaught of relentless and increasingly shameful attack of CSR? White answers it best:

> It is sad that this argument needs to be made, and if it were not for what appears to be a fairly strong commitment within the business community… in the name of the free enterprise system, the argument would not have been made… Unless we take strong and appropriate steps… society will be reinforcing a destructive mode of behavior that is maximally

95 Here, think of such instances as oil spills, tainted pills or defective medical devices, malfunctioning merchandise, recall of E-coli infected meat or veggies, or clinical trial catastrophe.

96 Get more at *PBS Newshour*, http://www.pbs.org/newshour/bb/long-legal-fight-bp-agrees-largest-environmental-settlement-u-s-history/. Viewed on July 9, 2015. Also see Margaret Coker and Benoît Faucon's report in *The Wall Street Journal*, at: http://www.wsj.com/articles/shell-to-pay-80-million-compensation-for-2008-oil-spills-in-nigeria-1420617029. Viewed on January 7, 2014. Also get NPR's online posting by Bill Chappell, at http://www.npr.org/sections/thetwo-way/2015/10/05/445983039/u-s-resolves-claims-against-bp-over-deepwater-horizon-spill. Viewed on October 12, 2015.

> disrespectful of human life, just as society would be reinforcing a value system that so emphasizes monetary gain as a standard of human success that murder for profit could be a corporate policy if the penalty for being caught at it were not too dear.[97]

In assessing the responsibility of groups, business corporations have received most of the attention. It has been so for obvious reasons.

3.5 Concluding Thoughts

In this chapter, I set out not to reinvent the wheel about responsibility which has bemused analysts from time. I set out to breathe some fresh air on it by laying the foundation on which to validate my aim for reconceptualization.

To sum up, if indeed it is possible to really sum up or arrive at any agreeable, quotable ending, having become more acquainted with the complexity of the different problematic aspects that have been touched upon in this analysis. However, several conclusions could be drawn. For one, individual responsibility for oneself is not being disputed here, it is taken for granted. It is also a given that all agents and entities, by virtue of their social existence, are (or ought to be) responsible for something or someone else.

The literary corpus on responsibility is obviously deep and dense, but of the much I have reviewed, I find quite a few of them enlightening. They include, Gowans' espousal of responsibility to fellow moral agents as being intrinsically and uniquely valuable; the obligation to be responsible for the other by Levinas; Gustafson and Laney's exposé of responsibility as an *ought*; or Richard Niebuhr and Bernard Haring's view that responsibility occasions a response or a call to action. Not surprisingly, most of these viewpoints may be judged to exhibit the trappings identifiable with virtue. They all emphasize the acquisition of moral character – an attribute that harks back to Aristotle, Plato but more truly the ancient Egyptian/Nubian mystics.

In effect, I have argued that responsibility can be viewed as a virtue. As a character trait or a disposition which is entrenched in its possessor, responsibility as a form of virtue, is a state of character by which, according to Aristotle, persons are defined. I extend this understanding to all 'persons' be they human persons or persons/entities in the legal sense. And just as virtue can be cultivated and habituated in persons with flesh and blood, so too can it be embedded or inculcated in the formations of legal entities in ways that are

97 White, p. 203.

action-guiding. As noted, the central question in Aristotle's virtue ethics is the pursuit of the good life for humans. Likewise, I don't see why that couldn't apply to legal persons, a.k.a., corporations or group agents.

For sure, this may be objectionable to those who propose the idea that corporate bodies do not belong to the moral community. But I'd insist that corporations cannot have it both ways. In their public relations, corporate entities seek to be reliable, even trustworthy, etc. These concepts, just like responsibility, are moral appraisals or normative notions by which entities are judged or assessed in the space of social norms. As I have stated, both the good of the agent and the good of the others, result from the exercise of virtue. I have also underscored the point that moral responsibility is neither contractual nor optional, yet innately other-regarding. As a cue to that, I presented responsibility in the context of virtue as a way of determining character ideal which lies beyond the range of self-interest.

In light of the above, the 18th and 19th centuries' Industrial Revolution perspective which saw corporations as legal establishments solely for profit making must be cast aside as moribund given where we are in the 21st century. It's about time to cast off the cloak of inhibition when it comes to making consideration only to bottom line; to continue to do so is to create a dangerous circularity. Resistance to that argument must no longer be made in subdued displays and lacking in conviction; a trend that is all the more mystifying given the abundance of obvious realities. Facing up to this fact is a challenge one would expect proponents of CSR to embrace, not shy away from. It's time we stopped pussyfooting around this issue; it is time to take it up by the scruff of the neck.

At a first pass, emphasis on profit making might have made sense during Industrial Revolution era when human conditions seemed to be receiving a new lease of life with new technological discoveries. But little could anyone predict some of the fallouts down the line. For instance, the likelihood that it could impede the development of genuinely shared moral understandings was beyond the raider. I argue that to insist solely or mainly on profit making is in fact retrogressive and signals a throwback to the worldview that modern society should be governed by "scientific-technical rationality" whereby success or technical advancement is measured only in terms of usefulness, efficiency and control. As such, quantification, measurement, cost-benefit analysis become the language for evaluating political, economic, cultural, scientific and moral questions and decisions.

The eminent critical theorist Andrew Feenberg[98] who is world renowned for his insights in philosophy of technology and constructivist technology

98 Feenberg, A. 2006. "What is Philosophy of Technology?" in *Defining Technological Literacy: Towards an Epistemological Framework*, Dakers, J. (ed.).

studies, has effectively critiqued this technical rationality which essentially is an instrumental view that rejects value-laden argument in favor of value-free or morally neutral view to our modern life. Defenders of this view – technical rationality – believe in infinite technological *progress*. In other words, the greater the technical control over nature, the better humanity is served.

Contrarily, and in agreement with Feenberg, the instrumental view that means are linked to ends or that technology always ensures endless progress, is wrong. Technology is not a neutral tool. Or we can look at it this way: the science of economics [production, distribution, and consumption of commodities] and ethics particularly, business ethics [the applied ethics discipline that addresses the moral features of commercial activity], are reciprocally conditioning; their shaping influence goes both ways. The tunnel vision which focuses primarily on profit making often lead to what Freeman Dyson has termed "revenge effects," that is, solving one problem while creating unexpected problems elsewhere; or an attempt that boosts profits to benefit a few people while wreaking havoc on a much greater number of people in tow.[99]

It doesn't need restating that without responsibility (legal, social, moral, etc.) no human society would be recognizable. Finally, I have argued in favor of adopting and adapting ethics into entrepreneurships by way of inculcating corporate social responsibility, stressing that to do otherwise would mean undermining vibrant capitalism (as well as socialism) upon which we all rely for survival. The argument that group agents or corporations do not belong to the moral community, or that they do not exhibit enough performative capacities associated with personhood to be treated as such legally, morally, etc., does not stand up to critical analysis.

---

99 Dyson, Freeman. 1997. "Technology and Social Justice." The Fourth Louis Nizer Lecture on Public Policy, Carnegie Council on Ethics and International Affairs.

PART 3

Personhood

CHAPTER 4

Re-Conceiving Responsibility: A Role For Personhood in African Thought

4.1 Introduction

In the previous chapters, my proposition to re-conceptualize responsibility in clinical trials took off on the bipedal themes of 'clinical trials' (Section 1, or Chapters 1 and 2), and 'responsibility' (Section 2, or Chapter 3). This concluding chapter starts with the presentation of the remaining part – the African notion of personhood. By adding on this last piece, my proposal becomes triaxial. As a capstone of this book, I aim to demonstrate how personhood (as viewed within the African communitarian/holistic backdrop), can fundamentally present a different equation when evaluating responsibility in clinical trials.

The challenge is to blend these seemingly disparate themes of 'clinical trials,' 'responsibility,' and 'African personhood' (full-fledge concepts in their own rights), to justify why it makes sense to couple them together for my purpose. The study structure and rationale therefore are cognizant of the need to establish the intersectional standpoints and the confluence between the three arms of the project. As a related matter, it is easy to misconstrue my reference to 'African notion of personhood' as essentializing. As I will make clear, I am not overgeneralizing. In fact, beneath the apparent diversity of African philosophical expressions of the self, there is a fundamental undisputed uniformity, thus setting the stage for a clear-cut cultural relativity (ethical particularism). As with many other African concepts, values seem to vary from one society to another, but in terms of their functions, philosophical grounding and interrelationships, some general unifying principles usually emerge. There is abundant literature backing up this prevalent view in Black Africa, and similar perspective in much of North ('Arab') Africa as well.

By introducing the philosophical dimension of 'African personhood' as a third panel to the equilibrium, I wish to provide a perspective of what responsibility can mean in an African context and then apply that understanding to biomedical clinical trials with human subjects. The overall analysis therefore follows through as the trifecta themes of responsibility, clinical trials, and African personhood, come to a full circle (see Figure 2). I'm therefore primed to adequately analyze the study thesis earlier formulated.

 | DOI 10.1163/9789004366947_006

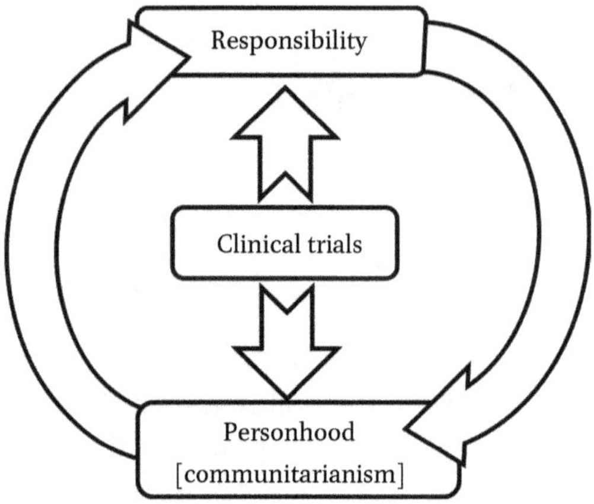

FIGURE 2
Dynamics at play.
FIGURE BY THE AUTHOR

Ultimately, this philosophical notion of selfhood will put in perspective my argument to re-conceptualize responsibility in clinical trials. While opposing individualism – a Euro-American mantra – the African perspective stresses communitarianism (a.k.a., holism). As such, responsibility for (and by) the individual can only make sense through the family, community, and environment in which he/she is rooted.

To reconceive and redefine responsibility, this study draws a sharp contrast between the role of selfhood or personhood in the Euro-American mainstream clinical trials arena and what I'd describe as a better responsible approach to clinical trials in the African context. While the human person has mostly been the prime focus of ethicists; how this selfhood is viewed in mainstream Euro-American bioethics practice is radically different from the rest of the world, particularly Africa. In what has thus far become the overarching theme in this study, the Euro-American emphasis is on the individual (individualism) in contrast to the African perspective that emphasizes the community (communitarianism).

Obviously, I am not simply claiming that communitarian (or holistic) view is novel. Rather, I claim that as the movement towards cultural diversity in global bioethics gathers steam, researchers would have to face up to the fact about this aspect of the African world view particularly on morality; essentially, that the devolution of the individual into his/her community is key. It is with this notion of personhood in African thought that I would suggest a reconceptualization of responsibility in clinical trial endeavors. Put another way, it is an understanding of the person from 'outside-in' rather than 'inside-out'; or the 'I am because we are' aphorism, that the reader can discern the full import of my exegesis.

As a guide, this chapter has four main parts. First, I will articulate in detail the notion of personhood by outlining and recasting some of its major features as expressed by a selection of prominent 20th century Africanist philosophers. The intent is to prompt interest and plot a path to understanding its multiple implications in bioethics (for instance, in clinical trials). I will demonstrate that in African philosophical thought, the concept of personhood is both pivotal on its own and on the collective bioethics project.

Second, I will compare and contrast the African vs. Western perspectives of personhood to highlight the stark differences and further demonstrate my preference for choosing one (African version) over the other (Euro-American version).

Third, I will parse through the subject matter (selfhood) within the bioethics framework. Though the concept of self has long been a well-worn path in Western philosophy and its contra opposite in African philosophy, I will strive to lay the foundation on which to extend the discourse to include the larger ethical questions that frame the emerging field of bioethics practice in Africa. I don't presume that all the necessary grounds and opinions will be covered adequately given the vast array of available literature and strands of viewpoints regarding the concept. I however wish to highlight enough areas and ginger enough interest within the limited time and space for this analysis. Considerations from relevant authors such as Godfrey Tangwa will help to explain and situate it in a broader context. While doing this, I will consider some general criticisms one could levy against the concept of personhood as found in African philosophy.

Forth, having laid out the logical premises, I will conclude by reconfiguring responsibility.

A brief housekeeping note: it is pertinent to observe that considerations of personhood[1] as an ethno-socio-anthropological subject matter can cross the boundaries of quite a few scholarly disciplines while assuming normative, thematic, descriptive as well as analytic tones.[2] Whether as a body, an embodiment, an identity, a selfhood, an individual, a human being, a 'man' or a

1 Person, man, woman, self, individual, human being, and to a lesser extent, identity, may be used interchangeably in this analysis to mean the same thing (in line with existing literary corpus). However, there are places where exceptions would be made or implied.

2 Some authors, example Polycarp Ikuenobe (2006), ascribe only two philosophical conceptions to personhood in African thought, namely, descriptive metaphysical, and normative. I am of the view that a more expansive analysis of the notion would include other related epistemologies and thus accumulate broader analytic frameworks and conceptions in the process.

person – objectivized or subjectivized – the discourse is guaranteed to be richly animating.

For analysis, personhood will not be viewed within a narrow confine such as ethno-philosophy – the study of collective forms of culture as manifestations of African philosophical systems. I will engage the topic as a concept in African philosophy *qua* philosophy. My approach will take the form of a second-order critical evaluation of first-order thinking within African cultural experience – a critique and revision of traditional African thought and culture. Nevertheless, I am cognizant of the vital role of other relevant areas of academic gnosis, for instance anthropology. To borrow from Ivan Karp and Dismas Masolo,

> Both anthropology and philosophy share questions about how the concept of the person is defined and used in social interaction. These disciplines take rather different approaches to the answers they provide. Both are concerned with distinguishing between the continuity over time that enables agents to characterize an individual as a "person" and with the epistemological problem posed by the differences between social attribution and self-knowledge.[3]

Supported by a plethora of conspectuses in African philosophy, the overriding thesis of this chapter sails on the fact that the African philosophical sphere, like its counterparts in other traditions, brims with familiar as well as not so familiar conceptualizations, some of which are yet-to-be fully explored. The list of empirical, ontological and metaphysical concepts is probably endless; they include (not in any order) the concepts of time, marriage, life (human, animals, plants, living-dead), spirits, God, nature, evil, justice, destiny, magic, and witchcraft. In both conceivable and pragmatic terms, each of these has notable implications for bioethics. But to deliberate on personhood in African philosophy is like threading through these concepts, such that a comprehensive analysis of it (self) amounts to touching on most, if not all, other concepts in tandem. But I will limit myself and make manifest that in African philosophical thought, the concept of man (or personhood) is crucially significant by itself and thus commands extra ordinary influence on the collective bioethics project (as can be witnessed through clinical trial lenses).

3 Karp I. and Masolo, D. (eds.) 2000. *African Philosophy as Cultural Inquiry*, Indiana University Press.

4.2 The 'African Man'

The understanding of the different expressions of *man* in African philosophy and religion may be pluralized, but essentially it is singularized. Less clear is precisely why this statement seems paradoxical; but it is not. Let me rephrase: African notions of personhood might seem many, but they are similar in their essentials, albeit expressed in different ways. This fact can be gleaned from relevant literature which posit similar or even identical depictions of what it is to be human in African traditional religion and philosophy. As we delve deeper, we shall see why this factuality should not be construed as essentializing (by way of devaluing) the African view point. It should in fact, be seen as a positive trait.

Also, I hasten to note that African philosophical discourse on just about any subject can rarely, if at all, be fully analyzed without adherence to religion or the spirit world, and for that matter, everything else (not to preclude atheistic opinions). African philosophical concepts are never considered as individuated concepts, rather they are holistic. For instance, it is common to see how an ethical discussion can morph into and encompass religious, social or cultural spheres. Take the concept of man as an example, the succinct words of John Mbiti (1970: 48) are handy here, "According to African peoples, man lives in a religious universe, so that natural phenomena and objects are intimately associated with God. They not only originate from Him but also bear witness to Him". It isn't surprising that Mbiti affirms staunchly that Africans are "notoriously religious, and each people has its own religious system with a set of beliefs and practices. Religion permeates into all the departments of life so fully that it is not easy or possible always to isolate it."[4]

In the oft-cited primordial text, *Bantu Philosophy*, the Belgian cleric and missionary Placide Tempels,[5] portrays man (or *Muntu*) as a vital force, a living being which radiates energy, or the being that possesses life that is true.

4 Ibid, 1.

5 Tempels, P. 1959. 1959. *Bantu Philosophy.* Preśence Africaine, p. 64. I will be remiss to not note that Tempels' work as a representation of authentic African philosophy has provoked mixed reviews. He has sometimes been a target of stinging excoriation and his work labeled as ethno-philosophy, i.e., philosophy deriving from the study of ethnic Africans. Tempels has particularly been singled out for pummeling and his work presented as having the intent to "colonize," "civilize" and convert the African to the "true faith." More charitable views however depict him as presenting a body of work that generally project the African as having robust intellectual and moral-spiritual capacity. Observations from both sides seem to be fair, but in this book, I choose to not take sides specifically because I am not critiquing his work.

It seems hard not to immediately notice the similitude of this view with the Judeo-Christian tradition.

> Man, is the supreme force, the most powerful among created beings. He dominates plants, animals and minerals. These lower beings exist, by Divine decree, only for the assistance of the higher created being, man.

Further still, the full meaning of man's life can only be realized in relation to other humans and the environment. This is a view that runs common among numerous other authors on the philosophical expressions of personhood in Africa (Mbiti, J. 1970; De Craemer, W., 1983; Menkiti, I., 1984, 2004; Riesman, P., 1986; Onyewuenyi, I., 1991; Owomoyela, O., 1991; Kaphagawani, D., 2004; Kelbessa, W. 2005; and Ikuenobe, P. 2006.).

> This living "Muntu" is in a relation of being to being with God, with his clan brethren, with his family and with his descendants. He is in a similar ontological relationship with his patrimony, his land, with all that it contains or produces, with all that grows or lives on it.[6]

By implication therefore, the fulfillment of a man's life depends on and is enhanced by the support and enrichment of all other life forces (humans/spirits) around, as well as other elements in the environment (say, minerals). In concert with this logic it is conceivable that a person's life's worth can either collaterally be enhanced or diminished by other forces and elements around. So beyond being a social being, man is suffused and suffuses in all creation. This relationship is so constitutive of the self that any serious disruption can lead to ominous damage to the person. And in the view of De Craemer,[7] the far-reaching relationship is therefore believed to be supernaturally, as well as naturally threatening and potentially destructive to the family and the community as a whole. Seen via the Bantu philosophical lens, the Bantu cannot be a loner. "It is not good enough synonym ... to say that he is a social being, he feels and is [in] intimate and personal relationship with other forces acting above him and below him in the hierarchy of forces. The human being, apart from the ontological hierarchy and the interaction of forces, has no existence."[8]

---

6 Ibid, p. 66.

7 De Craemer, W. 1983. "A Cross-Cultural Perspective on Personhood." In *The Milibank Memorial Fund Quarterly*, Health and Society, p. 23. But the implication shouldn't only be viewed negatively; in fact, it ought to be more positive than negative.

8 Tempels, pp. 68–69.

To further illustrate, let me borrow from the science of physics: if a person were to stand on a 12-ft stool in an open field, the fact that we can visualize him, i.e., detect his acuity, is due to the backdrop that spatially surround him. In other words, gratings of different waveforms and spatial frequencies make it possible for the visual system to measure the band-pass characteristics of the environing channels for the eye to pick out. In like manner, a person cannot 'exist' without his/her rooting in the surrounding community and environment. It doesn't get more powerful than that.

John Mbiti's analysis fittingly latches on to this thread of thought about which an extended citation is warranted here:

> In traditional life, the individual does not and cannot exist alone except corporately. He owes his existence to other people, including those of past generations and his contemporaries. He is simply part of the whole. The community must therefore make, create or produce the individual; for the individual depends on the corporate group. Physical birth is not enough: the child must go through rites of incorporation so that it becomes fully integrated into the entire society. These rites continue throughout the physical life of the person, during which the individual passes from one stage of corporate existence to another. The final stage is reached when he dies and even then, he is ritually incorporated into the wider family of both the dead and the living. Whatever happens to the individual happens to the whole group, and whatever happens to the whole group happens to the individual. The individual can only say: 'I am because we are; and since we are, therefore I am.' This is a cardinal point in the understanding of the African view of man.[9]

This person-community relationship is an idea that has variously been referred to as group solidarity (Menkiti, 2004); communalistic character (Wiredu, 2004); communitarian view (Matolino, 2011); eco-communalism (Tangwa, 2004); cultural collectivism (Schwartz and Bilsky, 1987); communalism (Ikuenobe, 2006); or communalism thesis (Kaphagawani, 2004). This characterization sticks out as the most outstanding feature in understanding man in the African thinking. I call it one-in-all relationship or bio-eco-communalism (BEC).

Citing two separate studies, Niehaus[10] makes bold the point that it is inadequate to view people in any typical African society as 'complete' in themselves

9 Mbiti, J. 1970. *African Religions and Philosophy*, New York: Praeger Publishers, p. 108.

10 Niehaus, I. 2002. "Bodies, Heat, and Taboos: Conceptualizing Modern Personhood in the South African Lowveld," in *Ethnology*, 41, 3: 190.

or as whole numbers without reference to other humans and the environment. This validates the traditional belief that each individual, or "dividual," is perpetually incomplete and is eternally being added to others, and is fully evolved after he/she is enmeshed and is meshed with others in his/her milieu.

Kaphagawani's[11] overview of the concept of person across a selection of West, East and Southern African ethnic groups, leads to three main characteristics of the human person: the force, communalism, and shadow thesis (the first two discussed above). As noted above and reiterated here by Kaphagawani who credits Tempels, human beings or entities "are nothing more than essential energies or vital forces. Force is not only a necessary attribute of being, but is (the essence of) being". Thus, Kaphagawani finds it useful to contrast the Western conception of being which is held static, to the African view point, which is constitutively dynamic or usually viewed in a processual continuum.[12]

As I have noted, the most outstanding of the three features is the one-in-all socio-centric view of personhood or communalism thesis, the origin of which like the force doctrine, Kaphagawani ascribes to Tempels and to a lesser degree, Mbiti. In this view, also noted earlier, the status of an individual is determined through cultural criteria or validation.[13]

Next, the shadow thesis seems to be the least on the totem pole. Credits go to Kaphagawani for his work in highlighting that aspect of the human being in Bantu philosophy that makes him "both a complete animal and a being with intelligence; complete because he or she possesses 'the vital principle of animality;' and intelligent, insofar as he/she 'is animated by a vital principle' which is immortal, and in which are anchored the intelligent operations proper to man."[14]

Further reflections on the concept of 'man' in the African thought reveal how it applies to the wider moral, juridical, epistemological, ontological and metaphysical realms. Given that 'man' as a force, does not exist in a vacuum, we are reminded that he is a force in the hierarchy of forces. In descending order, this ranked order of forces begins with God, the Great Force, then the spirits, founding fathers, the dead, according to the order of succession; then the living according to their rank in terms of seniority. "After living men come animals, vegetables, and minerals, which are in turn categorized on their relative

11 Kaphagawani, D. 2004. "African Conception of a Person: A Critical Survey." In *A Companion to African Philosophy*, Wiredu, K. ed., Blackwell Publishing.

12 Ibid, p. 335.

13 Ibid, p. 337.

14 Ibid, p. 339.

importance in their own classes."[15] Hence, the perceived bond between persons – an intimate ontological relationship – leads the African to know and feel "himself to be in intimate and personal relationship with other forces acting above or below him in the hierarchy of forces."[16]

Sequencing it further, African epistemology on man could be seen to follow suit by inference. "Knowledge or wisdom for the African consists in how deeply he understands the nature of forces and their interaction. [With God as the First Force and the ultimate wisdom], He knows all forces, their ordering, their dependence, their potential, and their mutual interaction. A person is said to know or have wisdom inasmuch as he approaches divine wisdom."[17] Thus, this proximity to divine knowledge is attained the older one gets.

The entwining of the realms of ethics and law seems to be the next logical point for consideration. Thus, the argument is that "An act will be accounted ethically good if it can be judged ontologically and by deduction be assessed as juridically just."[18] Viewed as both "metaphysical ethics in one sense and ethical communalism in another sense" it implies that the human conduct is always within the confines of a consideration for the community of vital forces whenever decisions of goodness or evil of his/her proper actions are being considered. Hence, all customary laws are therefore inspired, animated, and justified from the African point of view, by the philosophy of living forces, or growth, of influence, and of the vital hierarchy.[19]

With all of the above, it seems suitable at this juncture to consider Kwasi Wiredu's normative definition with a hindsight that ascriptions about personhood can be more than just normative, but also include descriptive, analytic and thematic.

> A person is not just a certain biological entity with a certain psychophysical endowment, but, rather, a being of this kind who has shown a basic willingness and ability to fulfill his or her obligations in the community. Personhood, on this showing, is something of an achievement.[20]

15 Onyewuenyi, I. 1991. "Is There an African philosophy?" In *African Philosophy: The Essential Readings*, Serequeberhan, T. ed., Paragon House, MN, USA, p. 40.

16 Ibid, p. 41.

17 Ibid.

18 Ibid, p. 41.

19 Ibid, p. 44.

20 Wiredu, K. 2004. "Introduction: African Philosophy in Our Time." In *A Companion to African Philosophy*, Wiredu, K. ed., Blackwell Publishing, p. 17.

This definition aims at the fulfillment or full realization of 'manhood/womanhood.' Ontologically speaking, we conceive him/her as an organism that has metamorphosed from the fetal to fully formed stage; having gone through a prolonged process of social and ritual transformation until he/she attains the full complement of excellences. And during this process of attainment, the community plays a vital role as catalyst and as prescriber of norms.[21]

A curious questioner might ask: are kids not considered humans in African philosophy? The short answer is, of course kids are humans. However, a more comprehensive answer will come in subsequent segments of this chapter, beginning with the examination of contrasting viewpoints between African and Western notions of personhood.

It needs pointing out that the fact that the African cultural settings are founded and sustained by shared beliefs, practices and values, *does not* make the individual to be inert or robotic with no autonomy and self-determination (as the individualistic perspective would have us believe). There is social control no doubt, but the apparent absence of metaphysical features such as voluntariness or freedom ought to be seen in the context that one cannot rationally act to meet communal obligations without recognition and validation of one's ability in pursuit of his responsibilities to the group.

Ikuenobe characterizes it nicely, "A person is not just an individual of human parentage, but also one evincing in his or her projects and achievements and adequate sense of social responsibility."[22] After all, "A community is a collectivity of persons, principles, processes, and structures that defines social norms, moral expectations, and responsibilities, on the basis of which one is recognized as a person." To not recognize this fact is to risk becoming a 'dangling' and socially disembodied metaphysical entity who cannot "apply communal norms to guide his conduct for personal interests and communal needs."[23] And to press home the bonding duty the individual owes the society, Heidi Verhoef and Claudin Michel[24] argue that an individual ought to contribute to the community not because it is expected of him/her, but because *it* [the community, *is* him/her.

21 Menkiti, I. 1984. "Person and Community in African Traditional Thought. In *African Philosophy.* Wright, R.A. (Ed.), New York: University Press of America, p. 172.

22 Ikuenobe, P. 2006. "The Idea of Personhood in Chinua Achebe's *Things Fall Apart.*" In *Philosophia Africana*, 9, 2, p. 118.

23 Ibid, p. 119.

24 Verhoef, H. and Michel, C. 1997. "Studying Morality Within the African Context: A Model of Moral Analysis and Construction," *Journal of Moral Education*, 26, 4: 389–407. The authors quote L.J. Myer, "Transpersonal Psychology: "The Role of the Afrocentric Paradigm," *Journal of Black Psychology*, vol. 12 (1986): 31–42, quote from 35.

As if that was not enough, here is how Theophilus Okere sees it,

> Man is not just an individual, an Island, left to himself and sufficient to himself, on his own. Man is essentially community. No one ever came to being as a bolt from the blues, like an oil bean seed falling from the sky, as our proverb says, I am always a we. We in the nuclear family, we in the extended family, we in the village and town, etc. One often hears of the vaunted 'rugged individualism' of the West… In Igboland, in Nigeria, in Africa generally, the community, the common good is the dominant reality and it alone ultimately provides the context and guarantee of individual rights.[25]

In clear opposition to Wiredu and Menkiti, to name just two, and in a move that signals a middle ground, Michael Eze, arguing against "consensus as a regulative ideal," apportions equal valence to both the individual and the community. To him, no community exists without its component parts; likewise, every individual's subjectivity is necessarily located and brought to fruition within the community. In his view, "To argue that the community pre-exists the individual is to argue that we can indeed have a community without a person for the community is necessarily constituted by persons;"[26] neither can you argue the ontologically contradictory opposite. Eze concludes that the identity or subjectivity of the individual and the community are mutually constitutive and that none is supreme. In other words, the individual and the community are engaged in a contemporaneous formation as neither pre-existed the other.

I admire Eze's efforts, but I think it will not lay the argument to rest much like the chicken or egg argument. Second, while I agree that the person-community relationship is mutual and constitutive, I doubt that it is *equally* so. Granted that the community is the sum of its parts; however, it is also true that the community can live on without one or some of its parts. The opposite cannot be the case, which is that one individual part cannot survive on its own for long.

I am more aligned to Okolo's[27] position which is that "It is the community that makes the individual, to the extent that without the community, the

25 Okere, T. 2005. 2005. Philosophy, Culture, and Society in Africa, Afro-Orbis Publications Ltd., Nsukka, Nigeria, pp. 3–4.

26 Eze, M. 2008. "What is African Communitarianism? Against Consensus as a Regulative Ideal" in *South African Journal of Philosophy*, 27, 4, p. 389.

27 Okolo, B. 2002. "Self as a Problem in African Philosophy." In Coetzee, P and Roux, A. (eds). *Philosophy from Africa*. Oxford University Press, Cape Town, South Africa.

individual has no existence." Put otherwise, though a community can and does suffer diminishment (but not cease to exist) when an individual part is excised; that isn't the case if reversed the other way around. Hence, I question the apportionment by Eze of equal valence to both sides. Nonetheless, while I concede that the community has some edge in exerting control, however, it isn't to the enslavement of the individual. There is always room for autonomous expression and self-fulfillment (something I have already noted above).

I am not enthused by the efforts of a coterie of Western-trained so-called African intellectuals (for instance, Anthony Appiah); and their home-grown backers (including Paulin Hountondji and Uwaezuoke Obioha[28]), who are influenced by alien literature and funding and would rather replace the time-honored African values and ways of life with some imports. For instance, they reject communalism on the basis that its emphasis on conformity, consensus, custom, loyalty and solidarity makes it constrictive of the individual liberty. They fail to see the import of the communitarian argument which is well articulated in Leopold Senghor's opinion that African communalism was founded on dialogue and reciprocity [and that] the group had priority over the individual without crushing him, but allowing him to blossom as a person.[29] It is by recognizing the humanity of others that one realizes the fullness of his/her own humanness. As we shall see in the next segment, the African person is distinctively infused in the African conception of the community and of the world writ large. The point made by Jensen and Gaie will soon be clear, namely that while Western notions of self tend to draw us inward 'centripetally,' the African notion of self draws us 'centrifugally' outward in relation to other people, the natural world, and the social environment.[30]

4.3 African vs. Euro-American Personhood

The notion of Western[31] personhood vis-à-vis African personhood is like night and day. Authors who have made comparisons in this area have commonly

28 Obioha, Uwaezuoke. 2014. "Radical Communitarian Idea of the Human Person in African Philosophical Thought: A Critique." *The Western Journal of Black Studies, Vol. 38, No. 1*, p. 13.

29 Senghor, S. 1965. L. 1965. *On African Socialism*. Stanford University Press, NY, USA, p. 5.

30 Jensen, K. and Gaie, Gaie, J. 2010. "African Communalism and Public Health Policies: The Relevance of Indigenous Concepts of Personal Identity to HIV/AIDS Policies in Botswana." In *African Journal of AIDS Research*, 9, 3: 297–305. 2010: 298).

31 I have applied "Western" or "Euro-American" somewhat synonymously in this analysis and the reason may be obvious. For instance, in bioethics, a field that took off in the U.S. in the 1960s–70s, it is clear that its philosophical principles are Eurocentric (deriving

singled out the Western perspective as the odd one out from the rest of the world (De Craemer, 1983; Tangwa, 2000, 2004; Tempels, P., 1969; Mbiti, J., 1990; Akabayashi, A. and Slingsby, B. 2003; Menkiti, I., 2004). But even as the Euro-American notion is the minority view, it is paradoxically the most publicized. If left as is, the concern seems to be that it is bound to globalize a less than global view.

A distinguishing trait you are wont to notice in many contemporary Euro-American settings is the quest and insistence to maintain one's own 'space.' It is a phenomenon that risks the danger of devolving into the narcissistic. According to De Craemer, "in present-day American society we conceive to a remarkable degree of the person in individualistic terms, emphasizing in this connection, his or her rights, autonomy, self-determination, and privacy."[32] In a twist that is laced with irony this has become the norm, despite the dominant Judeo-Christian tradition and doctrine that have for centuries been used to proselytize the need to love our neighbors as ourselves; to be our brothers' keepers; and even to love our enemies to the point of turning the other cheek when we are struck on one side. Yet, in the Euro-American tradition, filial relationships are highly restrictive, recognizing mostly members of the proximate (nuclear) family such as spouses, parents, siblings (and may be grandparents).

A review of studies on Euro-American personhood conclude that theoretical approaches on this concept present the person as "autonomous, propertied, self-interested, accumulative and having independent agency – measured in terms of its power of control over others. [The] individual's interest is seen as opposed to both the interest of other individuals and that of the larger social whole."[33] When viewed in this way, a chasm is thus created between the interests of the individual and those of the larger social group. There is even a

---

for instance, from the deontological theories of Kant and Mill-Bentham utilitarian principles). Further still, while bioethics is traditionally practiced in the West within the four-corner stone principles of autonomy, non-maleficence, beneficence, and justice; in other parts of the world, incongruities with these principles tend to emerge at the local level when their West-centric biases are subjected to closer scrutiny. Examples can be found in Akabayashi, A. and Slingsby, B. 2003. "Bioethics in Japan: The Second Stage," *Cambridge Quarterly of Healthcare Ethics*, 12: 261–264; DeVries, R. et al. *International Research Collaborations: Much to be Gained, Many Ways to Get in Trouble*, in *Normative Environments of International Science*. Anderson, Melissa S., and Steneck, Nicholas H. (Eds.), New York: Routledge; and, Diniz, D. 2000. "Feminist Bioethics: The Emergence of the Oppressed," in *Globalizing Feminist Ethics*, ed. Tong, R. et al., Westview Press, Colorado.

32 De Craemer, W. 1983, p. 20.

33 Piot, C. 199. *Remotely Global: Village Modernity in West Africa*. Chicago p. 18.

deeper divide when you drill the analysis further to expose pervasive logical-rational dichotomies.

> This view sharply opposes body and mind, thought and feeling, the conscious and the unconscious. Self and other, reality and non-reality (imagining, dreaming, and hearing voices for example are not real). Taken as a whole, our conception of personhood has at least one major paradoxical attribute. Although it places a high positive value on a universalistic definition of the worth, dignity, and equality of every individual person, it tends to be culturally particularistic, and inadvertently ethnocentric.[34]

Areas of commonality between the Western and African perspectives on personhood are at best marginal. For instance, both perspectives regard a person to be not just fully self-conscious but also rational, free, and self-determining.[35] Barring these, other aspects of the concept are widely contrasted. From all indications, the two viewpoints can largely be construed as contra opposites.

To return to my earlier point, the most prominent contrast is that whereas the Euro-American view of a person is that of an autonomous, lone individual; the African man/woman is far more dynamic and can only be defined by reference to the environing community. "And this primacy is meant to apply not only ontologically, but also in regard to epistemic accessibility the sense of self-identity which the individual comes to possess cannot be made sense of except by reference to these collective facts."[36]

The second point of contrast that needs reiterating is the element that a person in African thought is 'truly' a person after being through a process of incorporation – from birth to naming ceremony and several initiation rituals, to marriage and taking part in the regeneration of the human species. Thus, "personhood is something which has to be achieved and is not given simply because one is born of human seed."[37] Note that the question about whether or not only adults are "persons" in the African sense is partially being addressed here. But more of this can be found under the African Personhood and Public Health section of this chapter. Nonetheless, the innate value of each person is always intact at any stage of development.

34 De Creamer, p. 21.

35 Tangwa, G. 2000. "The Traditional African Perception of a Person: Some Implications for Bioethics." *The Hastings Center Report,* 30, 5, p. 42.

36 Menkiti, 1984: 171.

37 Ibid, p. 172.

These two traits, according to Jagers and Mock (1995: 153), unite under the communalist concept in the Afro-cultural setting that highlights the fundamental interdependence of people and expressed in terms of worldviews, sensibilities, and behavioral inclinations. Because communalism emphasizes the importance of social relations, it can similarly be expressed attitudinally on interpersonal levels. Hence, a communal ethos embodies a sense of shared goals, common destiny, and corporate well-being.[38]

Two empirical studies by Schwartz, and Schwartz and Bilsky,[39] strongly lend support to this thesis. In highlighting the polar opposites between the Euro-American and African conceptions of the person; they argue that in African culture collectivism emphasizes the promotion of wellbeing of social others, care and protection of kith and kin, sanctions against the violation of group expectations and mores, and a universal adherence to group customs. Conversely, individualists are groomed to be self-centered; accomplish personal goals; and, claim to possess unfettered functioning in pursuit of pleasure, sensuous gratification, and status and control.

On his part, Ikuenobe[40] is reputed to be unique in using an analytic methodology to reject individualism across the board. He argues for a communitarian state, for a freedom entirely constituted by communal norms and even for 'indoctrination' and 'epistemic authoritarianism' of certain kinds that he maintains are not merely innocuous, but also in an important sense, 'rational.'

It has emerged that the opposing conceptions in the two views (Western vs. African) are quite profound. Those divergences are here typified by Ifeanyi Menkiti's illustration.[41] As shown in Figure 3, while the African view allocates ontological independence to human society, and moves from society to individuals, the Euro-American perspective asserts autonomy and moves instead from the individual to the society.

---

38 Jagers, R. and Mock, L. 1995. "The Communalism Scale and Collectivistic-Individual Tendencies: Some Preliminary Findings." In *Journal of Black Psychology*, 21, 2, pp. 153–155.

39 Schwartz, S. 1990. Individualism-Collectivism: Critique and Proposed Refinements. In *Journal of Cross-Cultural Psychology*, 21; and, Schwartz, S. and Bilsky, W. 1987. Towards a Universal Psychological Structure of Human Values. In *Journal of Personality and Social Psychology*, 53.

40 Thaddeus Metz noted this point in his review of Ikuenobe's 2006 book, *Philosophical Perspectives on Communalism and Morality in African Traditions in Journal of Contemporary African Studies,* (2008) 26, No. 2: 231–239.

41 Menkiti, I. 1984.

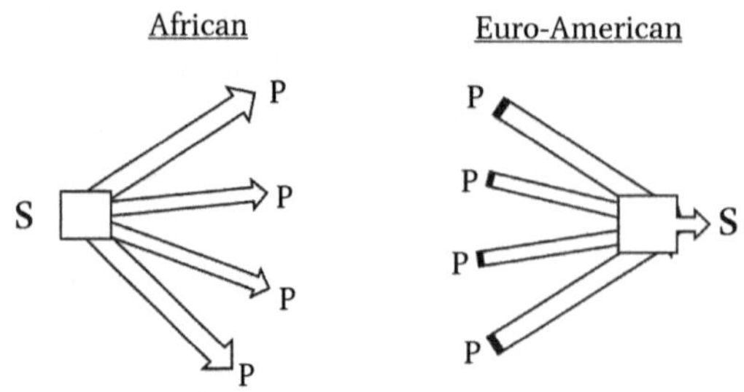

FIGURE 3
Polar opposites of selfhood (African vs. Euro-American).
MENKITI, 1984

The work by Godfrey Tangwa[42] further illuminates this African vs. Western juxtaposition, arguing that the Western conception of a person is appropriate only for the ascription of moral responsibility rather than for the ascription of moral worth. By contrast, the African perception of a person is drawn from the African worldview which incorporates all the categories and stages of a human being and intimately belonging to an eco-bio-communitarian moral community made up of moral agents.

Tangwa surmises that the Western ethical theory seems to concentrate on the *object* of morality, the individual, to the neglect of the *subject*, the agent. This he says, further conjures up the attribute of the principle of might is right, a characteristic of Western imperialism, colonialism, domination, exploitation and monopoly of commerce. By concentrating on the individual rather than the agent, Western ethical theory successfully shifts critical ethical attention from themselves and their actions onto their victims.[43] This, Tangwa concludes, is a value judgment that seems to be "dictated by economic considerations and the push for scientific progress and technological refinement. Science, technology, and commerce [thus] constitute the unholy trinity of engines behind the constant rethinking of moral categories in the Western world."

In creating a duality between the *object* of morality, the individual, to the neglect of the *subject*, the agent, many problems are kicked up rather than resolved. These issues have long historical roots. And not surprisingly, J.S. Mill might be influencing this thought process. In *Logic*, Mill speaks of things as 'non-substances' and 'attributes' as *objects* and appearing to "seek an alternative term which might lighten the perceived ontic burden, or carry rather less obvious metaphysical weight."[44] The nub of this suggestion is that for certain

42 Tangwa, G. 2000. "The Traditional African Perception of a Person: Some Implications for Bioethics." In *The Hastings Center Report*, 30, 5, p. 42.

43 Tangwa, Ibid: 40.

44 Read more in Stanford Encyclopedia of Philosophy (online), http://plato.stanford.edu/entries/object/. Viewed on October 2, 2015.

purposes, any implicature of substantiality ought to be detached, meaning nothing more than something, anything, to which one may be counted as one. This could as well be likened to Wittgenstein's 'pure concept object' which has no empirical content; or in a related sense the Aristotelian abstract and concrete objects.[45]

4.4 African Personhood and Bioethics

Who does bioethics? Everyone does it, but approaches differ (or should differ) mostly because it is conditioned by environing circumstances. Like politics, all bioethics is local. Put otherwise, even as bioethics practice is governed by 'universal principles,' particularism usually holds sway (or ought to hold sway) at the socio-cultural level. The principles of autonomy, beneficence, non-maleficence, and justice pretend to convey universalism. But in actuality, they can't escape from their inherent linkage to Western individualistic notions of personhood, in contrast to the rest of the world who sees the person not as an isolated individual, but as entities embedded in kinship, group and community.[46] Prima facie, it seems innocuous that personhood projects a universal notion. But under a closer consideration it is fitting to ascribe that understanding a relativist interpretation in order for bioethics to serve the multicultural interests of persons in myriad milieus.

Thus, it would be wise to heed the cultural realities and assumptive frame of reference of different peoples for bioethics to have any meaning. That is Segun Gbadegesin's argument in positing two aspects of a people's worldview relevant to bioethical issues: their conception of the human person and their conception of cause. In essence, "What [people] consider themselves to be and what they consider to be the principles of causation will normally influence their attitudes to health and illness and their choices regarding health care."[47]

Let me recap, conceptualizing the African person from 'outside-in' rather than 'inside-out,' makes for an exciting endeavor, particularly given its elemental dynamism. Though a composite and unique identity, the African conception of a person is vivacious; always in continuous process of waxing and

45 Ibid.

46 Get more details from DeVries, R. et al. 2010. "International Research Collaborations: Much to be Gained, Many Ways to Get in Trouble," In *Normative Environments of International Science*. Anderson, Melissa S., and Steneck, Nicholas H. (Eds.), New York: Routledge.

47 Gbadegesin, S. 1993. "Bioethics and Culture: An African Perspective." In *Bioethics*, 7, 2/3, p. 257.

waning in response to the play of forces within and upon its individuality from interpersonal, physical and supernatural sources. This communalist element and its deep-rooted effect can be felt in no less way than in health care. The individual is integrally located and anchored in a mesh of relationships within the family, village and clan (living and dead), all of whom are primordial sources of that person's physical, psychic, and spiritual wellbeing. This is particularly true of relatives or significant others, whose closeness may generate a host of contraposing attributes such as pride or envy, excitement or malice, likeness or hostility, love or rancor; and the capacity to harm or help through the harnessing of the shades of energy residing in the beings within his/her sphere.

Paul Riesman's analysis of issues pertaining to African mental health, child development and traditional conceptions and practices of handling mental health, provides one more inroad to examining this subject matter. The fact that it is common to think that your misfortune – sickness, lack of progress in the family, at work or business, etc., – could be attributed to other beings with whom you commune (people around, ancestral spirits, etc.), – can be a huge issue for public health. As a consequence, a 'group ego' conundrum is created which refers to the belief that someone "could be eating your soul or casting a spell on you." Seen as such the common African understanding of the person, which perceives the self as connected to forces and entities outside it, could present considerable challenges of its own.[48] On the surface of it, this attribute may be viewed only negatively or as a potential downside. However, doing so does not represent the total picture. Casting a wider perspective would reveal the overarching reality that African societies are organized around the requirements of duty and obligation to the larger community (as opposed to Western individualism). This broader spectrum makes for better understanding.

I proceed to test this reality with a health-related question: in matters of reproductive health and sexual rights, who owns the body – the woman, the unborn, the husband, the family, or the society? With empirical research finding as proof, Izugbara, C. and Undie, C. seem to answer assuredly that in many African societies, community fertility desires have been known to inform or, indeed, to override the very notion of individual reproductive choice both for the man and the woman.[49] This reality (justifiably) endues, in spite of numerous

---

48 Riesman, P. 1986. "The Person and the Life Cycle in African Social Life and Thought." In *African Studies Review*, 29, 2, p. 77.

49 Izugbara, C. and Undie, C. 2008. "Who Owns the Body? Indigenous African Discourses of the Body and Contemporary Sexual Rights Rhetoric." In *Reproductive Health Matters*, 16, 31, p. 165.

international declarations adopted by various (typically non-governmental) organizations and labeled along the so-called universal human rights.

The upshot here is that many of similar worldwide declarations ignore cultural milieus that are affiliated with strong community-oriented traditions; thus, resulting in incontrovertible tension between African ideas and Western discourses of the body and their implications. For instance, in African culture individuals (both young and old) reach their full stature only with the support and fellowship of their kit and kin.[50] This is the only way that the community allows the individual to indeed actualize himself/herself. Consequently, international sexual rights declarations – from abortion, family planning, sex education to sexual orientation – that are constructed along individualistic Western world-views, often result in tensive backlash in much of Africa. To reiterate a point that I made earlier, the African person is a "fractual" which cannot be expressed in a whole number. He/she is perennially incomplete and perpetually fused in the framework of a larger structure and built upon by the gifts of others. Together their actions are always in context and ultimate group objective is embodied in their dispositions.[51]

Let me reiterate for the umpteenth time: the strong allegiance to the community does not vitiate the element of individuality. If it did, there would be no recognition for individual's creativeness and inventiveness and which will lead to the erosion of human rights. One is not submerged in the group simply because he is a member of that group. His identity and interests remain intact. Yet, there is tacit de-emphasis in the cult of the individual.

In Oyekan Owomoyela's (1991: 157) exegesis, "The reason is not necessarily that Africans do not believe in individualism. Any society that encourages heroism and worships it, as Africans certainly do, evidently encourages individual excellence. [However] to attach one's name on an object or an idea is to assert exclusive claim and proprietorship to it, whereas traditional society frowns on the implied possessiveness and ostentatious self-importance". Citing Kwame Gyekye, Bernard Matolino (2011) reminds us that there is a difference between radical and moderate communitarianism, with Ifeanyi Menkiti representing the radical side and Gyekye the other. He affirms that "although there is widespread agreement to the fact that the concept of person in African thinking is communitarian, there is significant difference in the articulation of what that communitarian conception might be and the consequences attendant to such a concept."

50 Ibid, p. 162.

51 Niehaus, 2002, p. 190.

Similar to Izugbara and Undie's work but focusing on the HIV/AIDS prevention campaign in Botswana, Jensen, K. and Gaie, J.[52] point to how yet another foreign-conceived idea is force-fed on an African community without regard to prevailing indigenous cultural realities. More specifically, it was Botswana's wholesale adoption of an exclusive Western model of HIV prevention, testing and counseling program – an individual rights-based prototype – which negates the indigenous understanding of personhood or human agency as rooted in African communalism, and other existing ethno-medical beliefs and cultural practices.

The result of the prevention campaign has been insignificant if tepid in a country with one of the world's worst HIV cases (over 17 percent of the population aged 18 months and above was HIV-positive in 2008).

Similarly, Samuel Jegede (2009) has used an HIV/AIDS surveillance project as a case study to explore the concept of communitarianism. He concludes that "applying the Western concept of autonomy to research involving human subjects in the African context without adequate consideration for the important role of the community is inappropriate."

Akin to the recommendation above, Jensen and Gaie are of the view that it would serve the recipient community well if future public health policies or programs were designed and implemented with the realization that ethical principles or human rights norms are [actually not alien but] inherent in African communalist practice. Failure to, (1) recognize this cultural reality, (2) respect it, and (3) apply standard methods of research protocols, undermine mankind's ability and responsibility to control the HIV scourge.[53]

When communitarianism is applied to the public health sphere, at least two outcomes are immediately discernible. One, because of the interconnectedness and interrelatedness of human persons (and indeed of everything else in nature) whatever happens to the individual happens to the community in which he/she belongs. This is apparent because the individual is integrally located and anchored in a mesh of relationships within the family, village and clan (living and dead), all of whom are primordial sources of that person's physical, psychic, and spiritual wellbeing. By implication, if you are responsible for one, you are responsible for all (hence, I view it as a one-in-all paradigm). "An action is right just (sic) insofar as it expresses respect for communal

---

52 Jensen, K. and Gaie, J. 2010. "African Communalism and Public Health Policies: The Relevance of Indigenous Concepts of Personal Identity to HIV/AIDS Policies in Botswana." In *African Journal of AIDS Research*, 9, 3: 297–305.

53 Ibid, p. 302.

... relationships... in which people both identify with each other and exhibit solidarity with each other".[54]

Two, the African disposition sees health topics (wellbeing or illness) as a communal affair, sometimes to the point that the family (or community) has a stake in becoming aware of another's health condition and having a role in the decisions regarding his treatment – a phenomenon that conflicts with the Euro-American proclivity to individual right to confidentiality. This comparative analysis should be a teaching moment for researchers, clinicians, bioethicists, students and academics as they confront multi-cultural perspectives on socio-political and morality matters.[55]

We have already been made aware of a sure way to gauge the importance of the human person in African thought and tradition, namely the premium value placed on human reproduction. We are often reminded that children are so highly valued that procreation has always been the main reason why people get into marriage. "In [a typical] African culture, marriage for mere companionship is rare, if not completely nonexistent. A child is always welcome no matter how it is conceived and no matter how it is."[56] Circumstances involving taboos such as incest and rape that lead to pregnancies are routinely disapproved. But it's hard to find instances where pregnancies are terminated or newborns from such wrenching events exterminated. In addition, newborns are by and large, accepted even if they were born with disabilities at birth. Indeed, a human life is unaccomplished without a child. Ultimately, it becomes an integral part of what defines personhood.[57]

There is thus a meeting (yet contra-opposite) point of interest between the African view and these sorts of outlook with the assisted reproductive methods of the industrialized world for people unable to conceive through natural methods. While the Western perspective focuses mostly on people wishing to withhold, limit (temporarily or permanently), or eradicate the possibility of the individual's ability to procreate; the typical African cultural perspective is inclined mainly to aid the birthing of more and healthy off-springs (but would not hesitate to accept human infants even if they were born with disability) and to accord them equal (sometimes more) respect and rights as any other

54 Thaddeus Metz. 2010. "An African Theory of Bioethics: Reply to Macpherson and Macklin" in Developing World Ethics, 10, 13: 158–163.

55 Refer to Thaddeus Metz's review of "Recent Work in African Ethics," in *Journal of Moral Education*, 39, 3: 381–391, 2010.

56 Tangwa, G. 2004. "Some African Reflections on Biomedical and Environmental Ethics." In *A Companion to African Philosophy*, K Wiredu, ed., Blackwell Publishing, p. 391.

57 Gbadegesin, 1993, p. 257.

person. It is in this connection that biomedical or assisted reproductive methods will certainly find fertile ground in the exploration of the epistemologies of the cultural belief systems of the African.

The matter above immediately opens yet another point of disagreement between the African and Euro-American perspectives but which I'd rather not dwell much on. However, it suffices to note that while the African concept of a person is unitary, the Euro-American concept is critically bifurcated between persons and non-persons within the human species. As such, fetuses, human infants, young children, people with mental disorder, and patients in persistent vegetative state may be technically considered as non-persons, because they don't possess any moral standing in the secular moral community.

Tristram Engelhardt makes this strident point in *The Foundations of Bioethics,* a polemic publication that has shaped a significant chunk of today's mainstream bioethics practice. He makes bold to define persons as entities who are self-conscious, rational, free to choose, and in possession of a sense of moral concern.[58] Among other things, he assigns a 'special' status to the people he sees as human beings and denies same to "non-persons" who he says lack moral standing in the secular community. On this score, the African conception of person would certainly find it problematic (indeed, unacceptable).

4.5 Summary

I have presented a review of the concept of personhood as commonly found in 20th century African thought. Along the way, I have noted that of the different attributes that define the person in African traditional societies, what I have called the one-in-all trait, a.k.a. BEC, stands out. A remarkable perspective is here prompted – the communalist perspective which assumes priority in some sense over the individual in matters that guides right action, political choice, theoretical reflection and moral agency as the dominant approach when deciding how to enquire or act.

The African concept of personhood cannot be detached from attendant notions of communalism as well as socio-ethical duties and obligations and beyond the purposes of self-identification or justification. I have also articulated the concept of the African person as immersed in the various philosophical spheres, such as metaphysics and ethics (and by implication bioethics). In so doing, I think I have provided a platform on which to extend the discourse to

58 Engelhardt, T. 1996. *The Foundations of Bioethics,* p. 139.

include the larger ethical questions that frame the emerging field of bioethics practice in Africa.

Present among the numerous public health and biomedical scenarios across Africa are challenges besetting public policies and programs which cry for more articulate formulation and approach. I have thus tried to use the unique notion of personhood in African philosophical thought to bridge the bioethics discourse. This trend of thought is perhaps accurately supported by the argument that global bioethics will succeed *only* to the extent that it is culturally relevant. Therefore, bioethics must expand its vision. It is with such backdrop that a host of salient bioethical issues – including issues involving human reproduction, organ transplantation and biomedical studies with human subjects – can be hashed out.

4.6 The Die is Cast

Tantalizing facts in the preceding sections support the immediate move for reconceptualization. In terms of positioning, it's apt to gore the bull now that I have fully run the gamut and cleared the premises for my thesis. But for a quick reminder, here is the buildup. Research ethics principles grew out of the high value placed on protecting human subjects in research against a catalogue of biomedical atrocities of the past. This high value calls for commensurate high degree of responsibility for which the four principles were instituted to uphold. As I have shown, numerous studies have both extoled as well as lampooned principlism in research ethics over the years. It has been illustrated that while they might be more suited for bioethics practice within the Euro-American tradition (even with some difficulties nonetheless), they are not exactly so suited for other multi-cultural environments (to be exact, much less suited for the Global South).

The core of my reasoning is that we must restructure our philosophical platform more broadly and re-examine its implications for the future research ethics. Hence, I have proposed the need to re-conceptualize responsibility in clinical trials. My proposal is hinged on the concept of selfhood; more specifically, I recommend the African philosophical understanding of selfhood. This conceptual relativity has become exigent given the imposition of the mainstream (read, Euro-American) autonomy-based philosophical principles worldwide (but which have clearly proved inadequate in addressing multicultural ethical requirements). This is the case notwithstanding that personhood remains the pivot of the field. There is no dispute in the fact that the underlying focus or the main ingredient of bioethics practice (research ethics, in this case) is ultimately the human person. It doesn't matter whether we are laboring to establish thematic issues in medical policy, practice, and research, or teasing out ethical questions that relate to the life sciences, biotechnology, medicine, politics, law, culture, religion and philosophy; the primary task essentially pertains to values – human values within a given environing sphere. The objective of bioethics always involves sorting out the ethical tension between the social world and the persons who inhabit it. I am of the view that the multicultural challenges to the currently received principlist theory of personhood as a nexus for research ethics, is in urgent need for revision.

To restate, the Euro-American influence in the formulation of research ethical principles are borne out of individualism, whereas if we must be fair to admit multiculturalism, much of the rest of the world, particularly Africa, would take the opposing view. The four principles have met with resistance in other parts of the world where incongruities tend to emerge at the local level when their West-centric biases are subjected to closer scrutiny. The crux of this bipolarity rests largely with the philosophical conception of personhood (which in the African context, cannot be divorced from the perspectives of communalism, eco-centrism and even holism).

Given that the origination of mainstream ethics principles is Western and is founded primarily on individualistic terms, it goes that supreme emphasis is laid on personal rights, autonomy, self-determination, and privacy. In the same vein, it goes with theoretical approaches which view the person as self-interested, propertied, accumulative, and possessing independent agency with power of control over others. As a result, conflicts between individual interests and those of the larger social group are ultimately inevitable. In terms of ethical theory and for instrumental reasons, this translates to assigning significant emphasis on the *object* of morality, to the neglect of the *subject*, the agent.

Contrast that with my preferred version: the African philosophical version, which portrays man not as a self-interested loner who is obsessed with privacy, status and control; but a vivacious, unique entity who is ceaselessly waxing and waning within himself but more within the dynamic interplay of relationships with forces around him both on the physical and the supernatural plains.

I see the African self (vital force) as a being that is hooked on a grid. The energy that he generates serves his individual needs, but is also shared with other forces around him. But as the need arises, he supplements his individual energy as well with those of other elemental forces. In other words, existing as a power point in an interconnected network, he is a generator, a supplier as well as a consumer of the voltage energy of the distribution network. Note how the African man is capable of these interpersonal dynamisms due to his elemental attributes of being a vital force who is imbued and animated with a vital principle and above all, is anchored in the communal operations of other forces. As such, he is a force in the hierarchy of forces, habitually in intimate consanguinity with other forces above and below him. Therefore, the fulfillment of his life is predicated on the support of other forces (humans, spirits, the biota, etc.). Consequently, consideration for the community of other forces is always in the mix whenever ethical, juridical, ontological, epistemological, and other decisions are made. It is upon this platform that my reconceptualization stands.

Doubters might still want to ask: so, if a person is essentially community to the point that he is not just duty bound to contribute to it, but because it (that is, the community) is him, where then are his autonomy and self-determination? Well, I have addressed it by pointing out that the two are not contradictory – the individual can exhibit independence and voluntariness as well as attain full communal or social obligations. Indeed, it is by dialogue and reciprocity and recognizing the common good that individual rights are ultimately guaranteed. Anything short of that leads to one becoming a 'dangling' socially disembodied entity (physically and metaphysically).

I am under no illusions that my overarching suggestion about the relevance of ethico-cultural relativity, nay, re-conceptualizing responsibility from an African perspective (particularly for research ethics projects in Africa), is certain to collide with mainstream accounts within bioethics. Refuters of this argument are likely to question the rationale for 'erecting another layer of rules,' and whether or not it would change much, if anything. But a more objective assessment will recognize that the four principles are not an all-purpose set of tools fitting enough to sufficiently serve the gigantic enterprise of global bioethics. At best, it can be handy as a convenient lever that steers different value judgments close enough so everyone can keep their own opinions.

"There has always been an undercurrent of resistance to the individualistic, autonomy-driven mainstream orientation within bioethics, and that orientation has [largely] held sway."[59] I insert 'largely' because the communitarian orientation which has historically aligned with the goals of public health, has since become a force to be reckoned with and has effectively turned the argument on its head: the freedom of the individual can no longer be seen to always trump the common good or the public interest.

Hence, calls have been increasing for the balancing of individualism with a multicultural approach (communalism). This is because individualism has

59 Callahan, Daniel and Jennings, Bruce. 2002. "Ethics and Public Health: Forging a Strong Relationship." *American Journal of Public Health*, 92, 2:170.

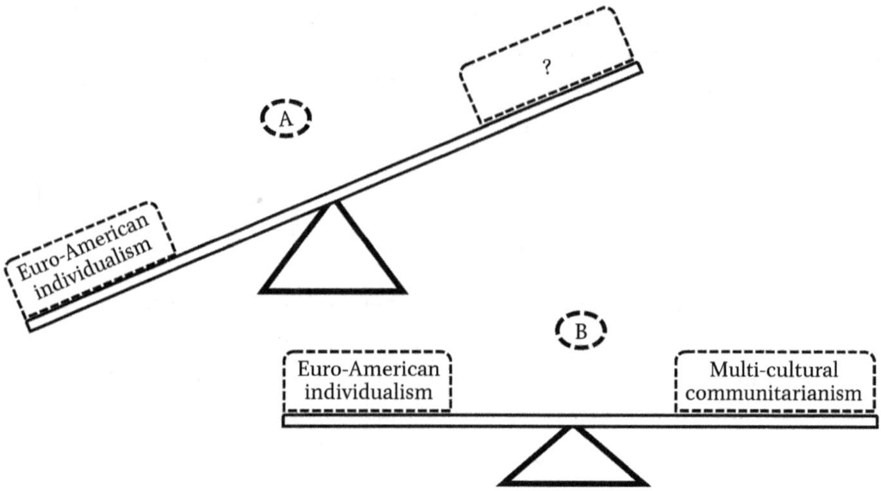

FIGURE 4 *Balancing mainstream with multi-cultural practices.*
FIGURE BY THE AUTHOR

been the view that drives much of bioethics today and weighing disproportionately in favor of Euro-Americanism (in Figure 4 above, compare Part 'A' to Part 'B'). In agreement with these calls, I aim to insert the African epistemology about personhood, a major perspective in African philosophy that changes the equilibrium in deliberations pertaining to responsibility for research subjects in clinical trials.

I argue that when clinical trials (much of which are currently conceived in the Global North) involve other cultures (particularly Africa – in the Global South, where many of the trials are often offshored to), there is need to frame and apply some additional considerations. The *status quo* has yet to properly formulate these considerations. As I have already articulated, the philosophical/cultural significance of the person in the African setting differs markedly from the Western perspective. I therefore see my suggestion to re-conceptualize responsibility from an understanding of the African perspective as a landmark point at which to address myriad bioethical issues one of which is responsibility in clinical trials; and providing a path to head off unnecessary philosophical, cultural and ideological tensions that are still lurking ahead.

The crux of my re-conceptualizing project, if it must be restated, is as follows: when communalist principle (personhood within the context of the community and his milieu) is applied to the public health sphere, at least two outcomes are immediately discernible.

One, because of the interconnectedness and interrelatedness of human persons (and indeed of everything else in nature) whatever happens to the individual happens to the community in which he belongs. The individual is integrally located and anchored in a mesh of relationships within the family, village and clan (living and dead), all of whom are primordial sources of that person's physical, psychic, emotional, and spiritual existence – wellbeing or otherwise. By implication, if you are responsible for one, you are responsible for all (at least in some degree hence, I view it as a one-in-all paradigm or BEC). Research ethics is right, just, proper, and culturally sensitive so long as it expresses respect for communal relationships in which people both identify with each other and exhibit solidarity with each other.

Two, because of this communal disposition, it follows that almost every issue with the individual is correspondingly regarded as a communal affair, sometimes to the point that the family (or community) has a stake in becoming aware of another's illness/wellbeing and having a role in the decisions regarding their treatment or upkeep – a phenomenon that conflicts with the Euro-American proclivity to individual right to confidentiality. This comparative analysis should be a teaching moment for researchers, clinicians, bioethicists, students and academics as they confront the African perspectives on morality.

Furthermore, I point out (with some personal sense of satisfaction) that the recommendations of the GMM project (see Chapter 2) directly boosts, without intending to do so, some crucial points that relate with my thesis (to re-conceptualize responsibility in clinical trials). They include the validation of the ramifications that are embedded in the centuries' old African philosophical viewpoint, namely the inseparability between humans and the environment (including human health and environmental health) as well as the interconnectedness and interrelatedness of all reality.

Notwithstanding that the transgenic mosquitoes' project as a public health intervention tool, had no primary human subjects, yet it is remarkable how it seriously considers the need to target the pathogens in a way that does not harm either environmental, or human health (plus, anything else in-between, e.g., the health of non-human animals and plants). In addition, it recommends that the overarching ethical goal in human subject research should be to respond to obligations to individuals being asked to participate, in this case, people living within the trial site who are classified as 'human research subjects,' as well as others in the adjoining communities being asked to host trials; while maintaining transparent and respectful channel of communication and protection plans throughout and long after the trial period. Thus, to accept the GMM recommendations, particularly the linkage between human and environment health, etc., is to commit us to the widely shared African philosophical perspective which expresses first, the intrinsic value of the human person, and the holism or interconnectedness – the unity – of the ecosystem at large. In its complete sense, this would cobble together both the physical and metaphysical/ontological realms of existence.

Overall, I consider the GMM's special attention to ethics and public engagement in public health research particularly remarkable in the way it provides for respectful manner of approach, the role of effective education and communication of goals and methods, and the provision of opportunities for follow-up discussions. That to me is an important element in reconceiving responsibility in clinical trials. As I have noted, the community engagement approach takes on a concentric relational web: from the core non-traditional human research subjects, to families, neighbors, communities, etc. at the research site. The outer spectrum recognizes individuals who do not typically fall within the definition of human subjects but who might be affected by the conduct of research in some way.

It is scarcely surprising that this suggestion lends support to the community permission model[60] that have long been prescribed by many authors. It is a model that requires *permission* and *approval* (my emphasis) from local authorities before biomedical studies are conducted.[61] As a practical, ethically appropriate, and common-sensical approach, deserving of any decent human endeavor, you wonder why it wasn't a standardized practice with a potential to eliminate or minimally reduce the chances of disrupting traditional social structure and customs of host communities.

My reconceptualization project is further aided by the GMM model for biosafety, ethics of engagement, etc. It thus reveals the need to improve the links between research and health care delivery and to promote the environmental, cultural, socio-political and economic processes that are involved so we can begin to widen our understanding of the vicissitudes of the impacts of public health research (or any other research for that matter). The GMM project, as a public health initiative, shrewdly recognizes that clinical trials ought to be applied within the context of prevailing social, cultural, legal, regulatory and political institutions. Couched within the philosophical commitment to evaluate clinical trials in terms of ecological and human health, the GMM project seems to rejig our thinking and thus spark a healthy debate. It does so while resolutely

60 I stand corrected by Paul Thompson who rightly notes that the two themes are not exactly the same. Here however, I am merely highlighting the support GMM's public engagement is getting from the community permission model.

61 One of the many suggestions to this model include that of Diallo, D. et al. 2005. "Community Permission for Medical Research in Developing Countries," *Clinical Infectious Diseases*, 41, 2: 255–259.

pursuing efficacy, transparency, responsible sense of purpose, quality and consistency in the process of testing and regulating new genetic technologies.

After several decades of viewing bioethics and environmental ethics as somewhat distinct fields of inquiry, it appears that our collective capacity to holistically understand and discuss these issues is witnessing a revamping of sorts. It is another admission of the inadequacy of principlism particularly in non-Western milieus. Also, it could be seen as a benchmark that clearly provides explicit and systematic delineation of steps for conscientious researchers doing work particularly in the Global South so as to make coherent the already widely accepted principles and benchmarks in international agreements or treaties including the Nuremberg Code, the DoH, and the Belmont Report.

4.7 Concluding Thoughts

It is a long-established fact that in ancient Greece (which is critical in shaping Western thought), philosophy was a search for the truth about nature and truth about man. In African thought (a philosophical tradition that precedes all others), it is about the search for the meaning of being, existence, life – all life in their order, interrelated as one continuum that finds fulfillment in the creator (God). At the fulcrum of that continuum is man, the center of all earthly life, all creation and in which creation is most made manifest. Thus, there is little doubt why the subject of personhood is both pivotal and zesty in African thought. Indeed, the richness of African philosophy can best be seen in ethics and metaphysics. "In these areas of inquiry, the concept of God and the nature of the human personality are the dominant issues. [More specifically], the concept of a person is probably the topic that has evoked the most interesting discussions."[62]

Advances in biomedical research exemplify the many strides in modern science. Thanks to clinical trials, these medical advances represent the unleashing of the human brain power in making his dreams a reality and in improving his/her physical, emotional, and material well-being. Sometimes though, scientific research has turned from being a quest for truth to becoming a search for material gains. This drive to dominate nature easily risks the domination of the human person along with attendant ethical problems – problems to which science has no clue, much less an answer. In this way, the very essence of humanity stands the risk of being compromised, sometimes irreversibly.

62 Wiredu, K. 2004. p. 16.

This book project primarily aims to reconfigure our understanding of responsibility in clinical trials from the standpoint of African philosophical notion of personhood. To accomplish this task, we must be willing to recognize that the West-centric research ethics principles have both been inadequate overall, and have continually presented incongruous dispositions in non-Western societies, hence the urgent need to complement them with other multicultural perspectives.

While I have not advocated a total renouncement of principlism, I have recommended the higher-order and more encompassing valuation of the human person (a point that both incorporates principlism but goes beyond it). In other words, I have not sought for the demise of principlism; but it's about time it either naturally metamorphosed, or is restructured into something better. I prefer the latter: rebuild the boat, plank by plank, while it remains afloat, to borrow Otto Neurath's simile. I have done this through the African philosophical lens of viewing the human person primarily with reference to his/her immediate surrounding – family, community, physical, and spiritual/metaphysical environment.

To sum up, I used the introduction to briefly lay out the trajectory towards which the rest of the work was gradually going to hone in on. For instance, some rudimentary questions were posed. They include whether science be left to continuously push its empiricist/materialist agenda unchecked. I also hypothesized that it seems about time to halt the Western extreme emphasis on individualism and the tendency to fuse, at all costs, knowledge and might, and truly acknowledge other philosophical and cultural systems. Then, I hinted about the tripartite thesis around which the work was going to revolve: clinical trials, responsibility, and personhood (specifically, the African notion of personhood).

In Chapter 1, I examined the 'clinical trials' theme both as the fulcrum of research ethics and as a concept that has endured since the dawn of experimentation, presenting a platform for analyses on a wide range of issues. That platform is probably more critical today than it has ever been. For instance, the 1996 clinical trials which followed severe meningitis and cholera outbreaks in Kano, a northern Nigerian city, that involved huge ethical issues with the American pharmaceutical giant Pfizer, provide both the catalyst and a test case for this book. But I am quick to remark that the citing of this case does not only serve to illustrate the imposition of the Euro-American autonomy-based philosophical principles on other cultures (particularly the African cultural milieu). It also points to the arrogant, ruthless expansion and exploitation of scientific and biotech markets; to the point that even the minimum that international research ethics principles demand was virtually unmet in the said clinical trials.

In considering this, I highlight the need for responsibility in clinical trials to be that character trait or ideal facilitating moral agents ('persons') in their professional duty to serve the common good while recognizing multiculturalism. Hence, I totally agree that when virtue ethics is "rooted in the narratives and aspirations of specific communities, [it] can particularly be helpful to professionals in discerning appropriate ethical conduct in multicultural settings and interactions."[63]

Nonetheless, as far as the history of biomedical research goes, the importance of the value of persons and the protection of that value, have never been in question. I have argued that the intension for which the now familiar series of guidelines and codes for human subject protection ought to be strengthened more than ever before, not least of all due to the impacts of globalization.

I argue that when clinical trials (much of which are currently conceived in the Global North) involve other cultures (in the Global South, e.g., Africa, where many are often offshored to), there is need to frame and apply some additional considerations. The *status quo* has not made provisions to properly articulate these considerations. As I have already enunciated, the philosophico-cultural significance of the person in the African setting differs considerably from the Euro-American perspective. I therefore see my suggestion to re-conceptualize responsibility from an understanding of the African perspective on selfhood as one way of addressing the issues and providing a path to head off philosophical, cultural and ideological tensions that have confronted, and will continue to confront us going forward.

In Chapter 2, I reviewed relevant aspects of the WHO-sponsored *Guidance Framework for Testing of Genetically Modified Mosquitoes*, which was proposed to tackle the twin scourges of malaria and dengue fever. The most outstanding aspect of this public health tool for me remains the unprecedented clinical trial protocol that it recommends. For instance, responsibility in clinical trials covers a wide range of ethics and engagement, community enlightenment and authorization in a concentric relationship. From the core human research subjects, to their families, friends and the community. The outer spectrum recognizes individuals who do not typically fall within the definition of human subjects but who might be affected by the conduct of research, either because they reside near the research project site, or that their daily activities and/or livelihood, including economic interests, could be affected by the research activities; etc.

The GMM's biosafety measures are equally ground-breaking in the manner that it plans for environmental safety. For instance, they suggest ways of

63 See Naomi Meara, et al.'s 1996 "Principle and Virtues" article in *The Counseling Psychologist*, 24, 1: 4–77.

channeling the experimental pathogens in a way that does not harm either environmental or human health (and admittedly, health of non-human animals too). These recommendations thus presaged the thrust for my reconceptualization project which I addressed in Chapter 4.

For Chapter 3, my analysis first took on the complex issue of what is meant by being responsible. For so long, 'responsibility' has remained a conceptual theme some theorists claim to have long shredded into tiny analyzable pieces and cobbled back. But regardless of this presumption, it however continues to challenge philosophers, neuroscientists and psychologists as they labor to understand our drives and motivations. In this book, I have not ventured to reinvent the efforts of other people; instead, I have tried to present a valid perspective in an unorthodox fashion.

I have noted that responsibility is a term that describes situations and actions involving moral agents or 'persons' on a day-to-day basis. In particular, it suggests as well as assumes a form of moral (social, legal, etc.,) obligation which we owe to ourselves, to others, to the society, and to the environment within a given circumstance. The obligation to be responsible can at times be formal, i.e., codified into laws as in laws guiding business transactions; as well as ingrained in the society's mores to guide human conduct, e.g., keeping within one's own without trespassing into others' property. In these instances, responsibility comes across as both a normative as well as a descriptive term.

Besides, I have also drawn attention to the fact that responsibility ought to be conceived of in terms of a virtue. In presenting an account of the virtue of responsibility, I went to great lengths to add impetus to the reasoning that goes with both individual and collective responsibility. I have resisted to be drawn into the sea-saw argument of whether or not we are responsible for our actions, to argue that responsibility especially that which is situated within the African cultural milieu, can help resolve issues that confront public health professionals and researchers. My discussion focuses on public health responsibility for certain social problems as well as how virtue of responsibility can point to what it means to act responsibly in public health (clinical trials). I have underscored the point that moral responsibility is neither contractual nor optional, yet innately other-regarding. As a cue to that, I presented responsibility in the context of virtue as a way of determining character ideal which lies beyond the range of self-interest.

The deep and dense literary corpus on responsibility that I reviewed include Gowans' espousal of responsibility to fellow moral agents as being intrinsically and uniquely valuable; the obligation to be responsible for the other by Levinas; Gustafson and Laney's exposé of responsibility as an 'ought;' or Richard Niebuhr and Bernard Haring's view that responsibility occasions a response or a call to action. Not surprisingly, most of these viewpoints exhibit some trappings that relate with virtue ethics. Like virtue ethics, they all emphasize the acquisition of moral character – an attribute that harks back to Aristotle, Plato and even the more ancient African mystics (in Egypt and the Nubia region).

In effect, it is easy to see how responsibility as a virtue runs deep in this analysis. As a character trait or a disposition which is entrenched in its possessor, responsibility as a form of virtue, is a state of character by which persons are defined. I extend this understanding to all 'persons' be they human persons or persons/entities in the legal sense. And just as virtue can be cultivated and habituated in persons with flesh and blood, so too can it be embedded or inculcated in the formations of legal entities in ways that are action-guiding. As noted, the central question in Aristotle's virtue ethics is the pursuit of the good life for humans. Likewise, I don't see why that couldn't apply to legal persons – corporations. Yes, if the primary pursuit (call it, pursuit of the 'good life') for legal entities is profit making, it ought to be within a social, not a self-centered context. I recognize that my position is unacceptable to those who think that corporate bodies do not belong to the moral community. But I'd reiterate that corporations cannot have it both ways. In their public relations, corporate entities seek to be reliable and even trustworthy (to mention just two). Both concepts, just like responsibility, are moral appraisals or normative notions by which entities are judged or assessed in the space of social norms. As I have stated, both the good of the agent and the good of others, result from the exercise of virtue.

To conclude the chapter, and given that the 1996 drug experimentation with children by Pfizer provided the stimulus for this research, I have paid close attention to the matter of whether or not corporations have moral responsibility on top of the responsibility to generate revenue for their shareholders. I have demonstrated my opposition to the argument that shields corporations from social responsibility merely on the claim that profit-making trumps everything else. Just as companies cannot engage in such questionable practices as polluting the environment with toxic chemicals, producing unsafe and lethal products, or lying and deceiving in advertising, so too would biomedical corporations such as Pfizer be held to similar ethical standards when they conduct research with human subjects, and to do so with sensitivity to cultural norms.

Finally, in Chapter 4, I introduced 'personhood' to complete the triadic themes by bringing to bear its African philosophical dimension. The notion of personhood in African thought provides a perspective of what responsibility can mean as it applies to (public health) biomedical clinical trials with human subjects. Ultimately, this move boosts my argument to re-conceptualize responsibility in clinical trials. While opposing individualism (a Euro-American mantra), the African perspective stresses communitarianism or communalism. As such, responsibility for (and by) the individual can only make sense through the community in which he is rooted.

As I have observed, when communalist principle (personhood within the context of the community and his milieu) is applied to the public health sphere, the interconnectedness and interrelatedness of human persons with everything else in the society and in nature are easily discernible such that whatever happens to the individual happens to the community in which he/she belongs, and to the environment in which he/she is situated. The individual is integrally anchored in a mesh of relationships within the family, village and clan (living and dead), all of whom are primordial sources of that person's physical, psychic, and spiritual existence – wellbeing or otherwise. By implication, if you are responsible for one, you are responsible for all (hence, I view it as a one-in-all or bio-eco-communalism, BEC, paradigm). Research ethics is right, just, proper, and culturally sensitive so long as it expresses respect for communal relationships in which people both identify with each other and exhibit solidarity with each other and with everything else in the environment.

Also, because of this communal disposition, it follows that almost every issue with the individual is correspondingly regarded as a communal affair, sometimes to the point that the family (or community) has a stake in becoming aware of another's wellbeing and having a role in the decisions regarding their treatment – a phenomenon that runs contrary to the Euro-American proclivity to individual right to confidentiality. This comparative analysis should be a teaching moment for researchers, clinicians, bioethicists, students and academics as they confront the African perspectives on morality. In the final analysis, responsibility in clinical trials is seen in terms of not only for the traditionally defined human subjects, it includes by extension responsibility for family members, friends, neighbors, immediate community, extended community, interest groups, the health and lives of non-human animals, and even the physical environment. It is a fallacy, indeed absurd to think that humans can exist or act as though they are independent of the environment they live in. Ultimately, we ought to see beneficence, non-maleficence, justice and respect for the individual's autonomy, as beneficence, non-maleficence, justice, and respect for the autonomy of everyone and everything around him/her (in varying degrees). In a sense, we are not just a part of nature, we are nature. In this way, the interconnectivity and inter-dependability, as well as the wholeness of reality are thus underscored, along with attendant socio-cultural, political, and economic ramifications.

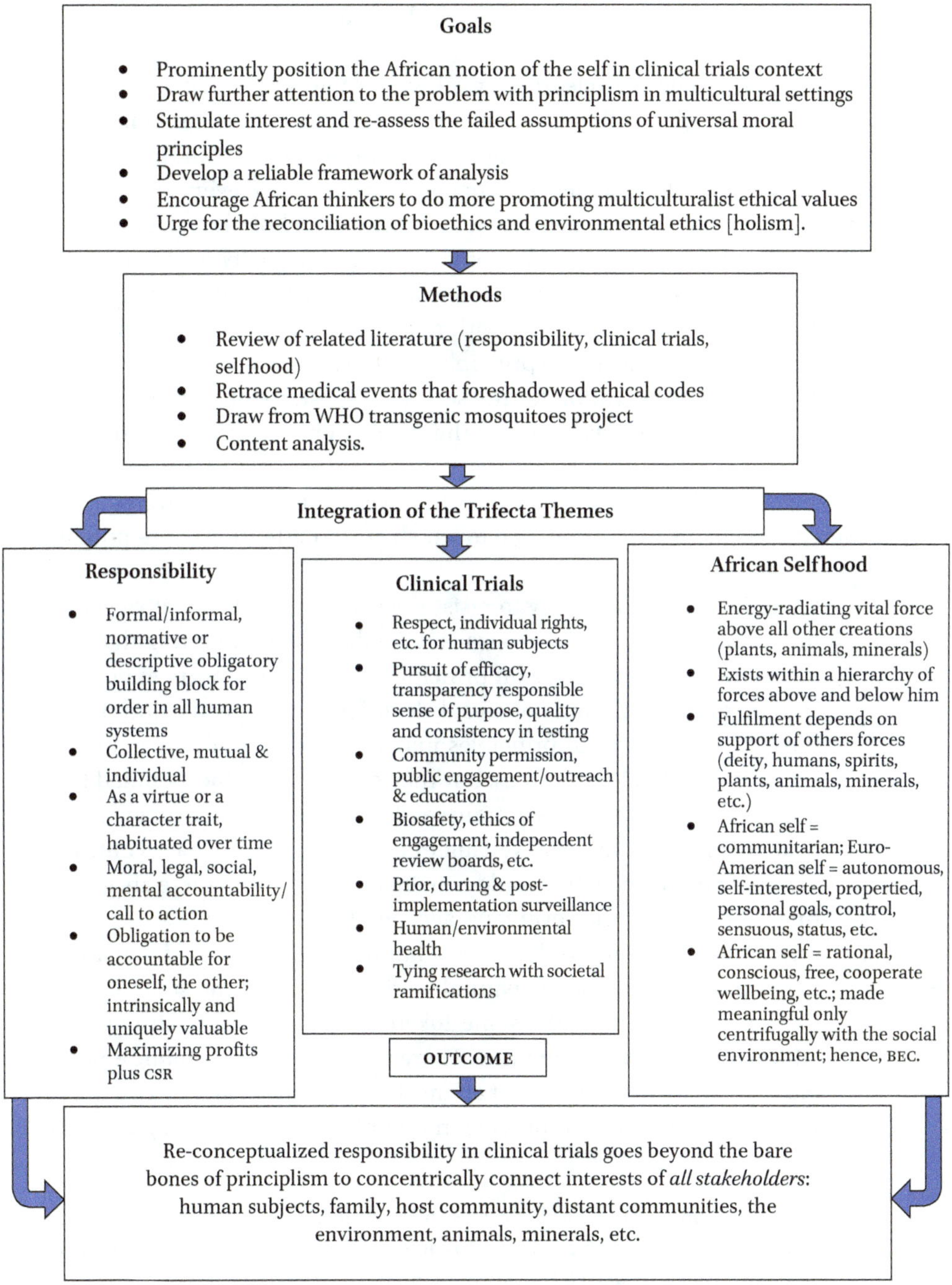

FIGURE 5 *Study summary chart*
FIGURE BY THE AUTHOR

4.8 Study Limitations/Directions for Future Studies

The focus of this book is clearly framed within the confines of redefining or reconfiguring responsibility in clinical trials with the understanding of self-hood in African traditional philosophy and culture. But, it couldn't have covered every aspect of the subject area or conclusively settled every matter in this regard. My analysis here is meant to join forces with scholarly discussions that have been gathering steam on the topic of cultural diversity in global bioethics. Hence, I align with the momentum which is aimed at forging an appropriate rubric for practice particularly with reference to Africa. I have argued that the autonomy-based bioethical principles are too narrow and urged for a more comprehensive consideration for the self – the substrate of clinical trials and the larger bioethical project – using the African philosophical insight about self.

Below, I identify a handful of topics that were either partly covered or not covered at all in my exposition, and to which greater attention are required:

1. I urge for relentless energy to resist the wool over our collective eyes on the question of ethical universalism. Evidence are mounting that even the Euro-American stance on principlism does not capture enough, including some subtle and not-so-subtle different European cultural structures. The basic ethical principles may function as reflective guidelines and important cultural values, but they can no longer be assumed to be universal everlasting ideas or transcendental truths.[64] More objections to Beauchamp and Childress' version of common morality have continued to find it dubious that "we could convincingly show that there are general rules of principles that 'everyone' accepts."[65]
2. Environmental health is the basis of human health. In fact, it is an axiom to say that the state of the natural world determines the state of everything residing in it. In the same token, environmental health ethics is ethics of healthcare or bioethics. There is a crying need to frame environmental discourses in ways that connect with public health discourses (or vice-à-versa) in order to provide more holistic understanding of issues.

64 Rendtorff, J. 2002. "Basic Ethical Principles in European Bioethics and Biolaw: Autonomy, Dignity, Integrity and Vulnerability – Towards a Foundation of Bioethics and Biolaw." *Medicine, Health Care and Philosophy*, 5: 235–244.

65 Kukla, R. 2014. "Common Morality and Embodied Practice" in *Cambridge Quarterly of Healthcare Ethics*, 23, 1: 75–85. I also credit my colleague, Dan Beck for calling my attention to this information.

For instance, the clinical trials process can never be sufficiently made meaningful without reference to environmental ramifications (be they physical, social, or spiritual). Part of my analysis in Chapter 2 point to this self-evident fact but a lot more needs to be done.

3. In many African settings (rural and urban), traditional medicine has played a significant role in the healthcare delivery going back to ancient times. More recently it has complemented the modern medical practice. But it is almost inconceivable to put in the same bucket list the modern form of clinical trial protocols along with traditional medicine practice. However, it would be worth the effort to elevate the notion of self in indigenous biomedical practice and discourse by researching it further. Thus, examining this notion in the traditional medical practice will contribute, authenticate, and further elevate African values by highlighting many of its unexplored dimensions. It will also help to articulate its theoretical basis and render research in indigenous medicine more ethically grounded.

Bibiliography

Akabayashi, A. and B. Slingsby. 2003. "Bioethics in Japan: The Second Stage," Cambridge Quarterly of Healthcare Ethics 12 (2003): 261–264. doi: 10.1017/S0963180103123079.

Amundsen, Darrel. 1981. "Casuistry and Professional Obligations: The Regulation of Physicians by the Court of Conscience in the Middle Ages." Transactions and Studies of the College Physicians of Philadelphia, Part 1, Series 5, 3 no. 22 (1981): 34–35.

Anderson, Susan. "Being Morally Responsible for an Action Versus Acting Responsibly or Irresponsibly." Journal of Philosophical Research 20 (1995): 453–462.

Andre, Judy. *Bioethics as Practice*. North Carolina: The University of North Carolina Press, 2002.

Annas, Julia. *The Morality of Happiness*. New York: Oxford University Press, 1993.

Aristotle. *Nicomachean Ethics,* with translation by W.D. Ross, 350 B.C.E. http://classics.mit.edu/Aristotle/nicomachaen.2.ii.html.

Asante, Molefi. *The Egyptian Philosophers: Ancient African Voices from Imhotep to Akhenaten*. Chicago: African American Images, 2000.

Audi, Robert. "Reliability as a Virtue." Philosophical Studies 142 (2009): 43–54.

Barry, Michele and Malcolm Molyneux. "Ethical Dilemmas in Malaria Drug and Vaccine Trials: A Bioethical Perspective." Journal of Medical Ethics 18 (1992): 189–192.

Beauchamp, Tom and James Childress. *Principles of Biomedical Ethics*, 7th edition; NY: Oxford University Press, 2012.

Benatar, Solomon. "Rationally Defensible Standards for Research in Developing Countries." Health and Human Rights: An International Journal 8, no. 1(2004): 197–202.

Bierhoff, Hans-Werner and Ann Auhagen. "Responsibility as a Fundamental Phenomenon." In Responsibility: The Many Faces of a Social Phenomenon, edited by Ann Auhagen and Hans-Werner, 1–8. London: Routledge, 2001.

Birnbacher, Diater. "Philosophical Foundations of Responsibility." In Responsibility: The Many Faces of a Social Phenomenon, edited by Ann Auhagen and Hans-Werner, 1–8. London: Routledge, 2001.

Boxer, Karin. *Rethinking Responsibility*. Oxford: Oxford University Press, 2013.

Bren, Linda. *Frances Oldham Kelsey: FDA Medical Reviewer Leaves Her Mark on History*, FDA Consumer Magazine, 35, 2001. https://permanent.access.gpo.gov/lps1609/www.fda.gov/fdac/features/2001/201_kelsey.html.

Bynum, William. "Reflections on the History of Human Experimentation." In the Use of Human Beings in Research, edited by Stuart Spicker, Ilai Alon, Andre de Vries, Tristram Engelhardt Jr., 29–46. Kluwer Academic Publishers, 1988.

Cafaro, Philip. *Virtue Ethics (Not Too) Simplified*. Theoretical Ethics, Southwest State University, last modified December 10, 2017, http://www.bu.edu/wcp/Papers/TEth/TEthCafa.htm.

Cahn, S. *Seven Masterpieces of Philosophy*. New York: Pearson Longman, 2008.

Callahan, Daniel and Bruce Jennings. "Ethics and Public Health: Forging a Strong Relationship." American Journal of Public Health 92, no. 2 (2002): 170. doi: 10.2105/AJPH.92.2.169.

Carpentier, Richard. Why is Research Subjects Protection in International Research So Important Now? Presentation on theme: "International Research and Subjects Protections, National Council on Ethics in Human Research and FOCUS Secretariat, CANADA," 2001, last modified December 15, 2017. http://slideplayer.com/slide/1686482/.

Coker, Margaret and Benoît Faucon, "Shell to Pay $80 Million Compensation for Oil Spills in Nigeria." The Wall Street Journal (New York, NY), last modified Jan. 7, 2015. http://www.wsj.com/articles/shell-to-pay-80-million-compensation-for-2008-oil-spills-in-nigeria-1420617029.

Coleman, Carl H.; Jerry A. Menikoff; Jesse A. Goldner; and Nancy N Dubler. *The Ethics and Regulation of Research with Human Subjects: Teachers' Manual*, New Jersey: Matthew Bender and Company, Inc., 2005.

Crisp, Roger. "Modern Moral Philosophy and the Virtues." In How Should One Live? Essays on the Virtues, edited by Roger Crisp 1–18. Oxford: Oxford University Press, 1996.

Dancy, Jonathan. *Moral Reasons*. Cambridge, Massachusetts: Blackwell, 1993.

De Craemer, Willy. "A Cross-Cultural Perspective on Personhood." The Milibank Memorial Fund Quarterly. Health and Society 61, no. 1 (1983): 19–34.

De Vries, R., L.M. Rott, & Y. Paruchuri "International Research Collaborations: Much to be Gained, Many Ways to Get in Trouble." In Normative Environments of International Science, edited by Melissa Anderson and Nicholas Steneck, 105–120. New York: Routledge, 2010.

Diallo, Dapa; Doumbo Ogobara; Christopher Plowe; Thomas Wellems; Ezekiel Emmanuel; Samia Hurst. "Community Permission for Medical Research in Developing Countries." Clinical Infectious Diseases 41, no. 2 (2005): 255–259. doi: 10.1086/430707.

Dickerson, Caitlin. "Secret World War II Chemical Experiments Tested Troops by Race." *National Public Radio*, last modified June 22, 2015a. http://www.npr.org/2015/06/22/415194765/u-s-troops-tested-by-race-in-secret-world-war-ii-chemical-experiments.

Dickerson, Caitlin. "The VA's Broken Promise to Thousands of Vets Exposed to Mustard Gas." *National Public Radio*. June 22, 2015b. http://www.npr.org/2015/06/23/416408655/the-vas-broken-promise-to-thousands-of-vets-exposed-to-mustard-gas.

Diniz, Debora and Ana Gonzalez. "Feminist Bioethics: The Emergence of the Oppressed." In Globalizing Feminist Ethics, edited by Rosemary Tong, 62–72. Colorado: Westview Press, 2001.

Diop, Cheikh. *The African Origin of Civilization: Myth or Reality*. Chicago: Lawrence Hill & Co, 1974.

Dyson, Freeman. "Technology and Social Justice." The Fourth Louis Nizer Lecture on Public Policy; Carnegie Council on Ethics and International Affairs, 1997.

Egbeke, A. (other bibliographical entries missing), 2006.

El Setouhy, Maged. et al. "Moral Standards for Research in Developing Countries from 'Reasonable Availability' to 'Fair Benefits'" The Hastings Center Report 34, no. 3 (2004): 17–27.

Elliot, Kevin. *Is a Little Pollution Good for You?* New York: Oxford University Press, 2011.

Emanuel, Ezekiel, David Wendler, Jack Killen, Christine Grady. 2004. "What Makes Clinical Research in Developing Countries Ethical? The Benchmarks of Ethical Research." The Journal of Infectious Diseases 189, no. 5 (2004): 930–937.

Engelhardt, Tristram. *The Foundations of Bioethics*, New York: Oxford University Press, 1996.

Eze, Onyebuchi. "What is African Communitarianism? Against Consensus as a Regulative Ideal." South African Journal of Philosophy 27, no. 4 (2008): 386–399.

Federal Ministry of Health, Abuja, Nigeria. "Report of an Investigation Committee on the Clinical Trial of Trovafloxacin (Trovan) by Pfizer, Kano, 1996." 1–83, 2001.

Feenberg, Andrew. "What is Philosophy of Technology?" In Defining Technological Literacy: Towards an Epistemological Framework, edited by John Dakers, 5–16. England: Palgrave Macmillan, 2006.

Feinberg, Joel. *Collective Responsibility: Doing and Deserving: Essays in the Theory of Responsibility,* Princeton: Princeton University Press, 1970.

Fitzgerald, Daniel and Angela Wasunna. "Away from Exploitation and Towards Engagement: An Ethical Compass for Medical Researchers Working in Resource-Poor Countries." The Journal of Law, Medicine & Ethics; 33, no. 3 (2005): 559–565.

Fitzgerald, Daniel, Angela Wasunna, Jean Pape. "Ten Questions Institutional Review Boards Should Ask When Reviewing International Clinical Research Protocols." The Hastings Center 25, no. 2 (2003): 14–18.

French, Peter. "The Corporation as a Moral Person." In Collective Responsibility: Five Decades of Debate in Theoretical and Applied Ethics, edited by Larry May and Stacey Hoffman. Maryland: Rowman & Littlefield Publishers, Inc., 1991.

Gbadegesin, Segun. "Bioethics and Culture: An African Perspective." Bioethics 7 no. 2–3 (1993): 257–262. doi: 10.1111/j.1467-8519.1993.tb00292.x.

Gowans, Christopher. *Innocence Lost: An Examination of Inescapable Moral Wrongdoing*. New York: Oxford University Press, 1994.

Greco, John. *Putting Skeptics in Their Place: The Nature of Skeptical Arguments and Their Role in Philosophical Inquiry*. Cambridge: Cambridge University Press, 2000.

Greco, John. (Ed.). *Ernest Sosa and His Critics*. Oxford: Blackwell Publishing, 2004.

Gustafson, James and James Laney (Eds.). *On Being Responsible: Issues in Personal Ethics*. New York: Harper & Row, Publishers, 1968.

Hager, Mark. "Bodies Politic: The Progressive History of Organizational 'Real Entity' Theory." University of Pittsburg Law Review 50 (1988): 575–654.

Held, Virginia. "Can a Random Collective be Morally Responsible?" Journal of Philosophy 67 (1970): 471–481.

Hicks, Stephen. 2009. "What Business Ethics Can Learn from Entrepreneurship," The Journal of Private Enterprise 24 no. 2 (2009): 49–57.

Hinde, Robert. 2001. "Responsibility: A Biological Perspective." In Responsibility: The Many Faces of a Social Phenomenon, edited by Ann Auhagen and Hans-Werner Bierhoff, 23–34. London: Routledge, 2001.

Hyder, A.A., S.A. Wali, A.N. Khan, N.B. Teoh, N.E. Kass, and L. Dawson "Ethical Review of Health Research: A Perspective from Developing Country Researchers." Journal of Medical Ethics, 30, no. 1 (2004): 68–72.

Ikuenobe, Polycarp. "The Idea of Personhood in Chinua Achebe's *Things Fall Apart*." Philosophia Africana 9 no. 2 (2006a): 117–131.

Ikuenobe, Polycarp. *Philosophical Perspectives on Communalism and Morality in African Traditions*, Lexington Books, Oxford, UK, 2006b.

Imran, Sophia; Khorshed Alam; and Narelle Beaumont. "Reinterpreting the Definition of Sustainable Development for a More Ecocentric Reorientation." Sustainable Development No. 22 (2014): 134–144.

Ingwe, Richard; Joseph Ebegbulem and C. Ikeji "Ecocentric and Anthropocentric Policies and Crises in Climate/environment, Finance and Economy: Implications of the Emerging Green Policy of the Obama Administration for Africa's Sustainable Development." African Journal of Political Science and International Relations 4 no. 1 (2010): 1–012.

International Conference on Harmonization of Technical Requirements, for Registration of Pharmaceuticals for Human Use, ICH, "Harmonized Tripartite Guideline for Good Clinical Practice E6(R1)," Step 4 version, 1996.

Internet Encyclopedia of Philosophy. "The Origin of the Notion of Bioethics." http://www.iep.utm.edu/bioethic/#SH2a.

Irving, Dianne. "What is 'Bioethics' (Quid est 'Bioethics'?") Unpublished Essay. Tenth Annual Conference: Life and Learning X (in press), Washington, DC: University Faculty for Life, Georgetown University, 2000.

Izugbara, Chimaroke and Chi-Chi Undie. "Who Owns the Body? Indigenous African Discourses of the Body and Contemporary Sexual Rights Rhetoric." Reproductive Health Matters 16 no. 31 (2008): 159–167.

Jackson, Robert. "Report of Robert H. Jackson to the President." Department of State Bulletin, June 10, 1945, last modified November 15, 22, 2014. http://www.ibiblio.org/pha/war.term/trib_07.html.

Jagers, Robert and Lynne Mock. "The Communalism Scale and Collectivistic-Individual Tendencies: Some Preliminary Findings." Journal of Black Psychology 21 no. 2 (1995): 153–167.

Jegede, Samuel. 2009. "African Ethics, Health Care Research and Community and Individual Participation." Journal of Asian and African Studies 44 (2009): 239.

Jensen, Kipton and Joseph Gaie. 2010. "African Communalism and Public Health Policies: The Relevance of Indigenous Concepts of Personal Identity to HIV/AIDS Policies in Botswana." African Journal of AIDS Research 9 no. 3 (2010): 297–305.

Jercker, Nancy; Albert Jonsen and Robert Pearlman. *Bioethics: An Introduction to the History, Methods and Practice.* Boston: Jones & Bartlett Publishers, 1997.

Jonas, Hans. "Technology and Responsibility: The Ethics of an Endangered Future." In Responsibilities to Future Generations, New York: Prometheus Books, 1981.

Jonsen, Albert. *The Birth of Bioethics*. New York: Oxford University Press, 1998.

Karp, Ivan and D Masolo. *African Philosophy as Cultural Inquiry*, Indiana University Press, 2000.

Kaphagawani, Diddier. "African Conception of a Person: A Critical Survey." In A Companion to African Philosophy, edited by Kwasi Wiredu, 332–342. Blackwell Publishing, 2004. doi: 10.1002/9780470997154.ch26.

Kass, N., L. Dawson, & N.I. Loyo-Berrios "Ethical Oversight of Research in Developing Countries." Ethics and Human Research. The Hastings Center 25 no. 2 (2003): 1–10.

Kelbessa, Workineh. 2005a. "The Utility of Ethical Dialogue for Marginalized Voices in Africa." Department of Philosophy, Addis Ababa University, P.O. Box 150012, Addis Ababa, Ethiopia, last modified December 16, 2017. http://pubs.iied.org/pdfs/13508IIED.pdf?.

Kelbessa, Workineh. "Indigenous Environmental Philosophy." In The Oxford Handbook of World Philosophy, edited by William Edelglass and Jay L. Garfield, 574–581. Oxford: Oxford University Press, Inc., 2011a. doi:10.1093/oxfordhb/9780195328998.003.0049.

Kelbessa, Workineh. "Indigenous and Modern Environmental Ethics: A Study of the Indigenous Oromo Environmental Ethic and Modern Issues of Environment and Development." Washington DC: Cultural Heritage and Contemporary Change, Series II, Africa 13, 2011b.

Kelbessa, Workineh. "The Utility of Ethical Dialogue for Marginalized Voices in Africa." 2005b. (Other citation details missing).

Khoury, Muin. "Genetic Epidemiology and the Future of Disease Prevention and Public Health." Epidemiology Reviews, 19 no. 1 (1997): 176.

Kiadó, Akadémiai. "Theory of Complex Environmental Responsibility." Társadalomkutatás 29 no. 3 (2011): 303–314.

King, Matt. "K.E. Boxer's *Rethinking Responsibility*." UCLA School of Law, last modified, December 12, 2017. https://ndpr.nd.edu/news/42145-rethinking-responsibility/.

Kukla, Rebecca. "Living with Pirates: Common Morality and Embodied Practice." Cambridge Quarterly of Healthcare Ethics 23 no. (2014): 75–85. doi:10.1017/S0963180113000480.

Ladd, John. "Morality and the Ideal of Rationality in Formal Organizations." *The Monist* 54 no. 4 (1970): 488–516.

Leopold, Waldo. *A Sand County Almanac*, Oxford: Oxford University Press, 1949.

Levinas, Emmanuel. *Ethics and Infinity*. Pittsburg: Duquesne University Press, 1985.

Light, Andrew and Holmes Rolston (Eds.). *Environmental Ethics: An Anthology*, Massachusetts: Blackwell Publishers Ltd., 2003.

List, Christian and Philip Pettit. *Group Agency: The Possibility, Design, and Status of Corporate Agents*. Oxford: Oxford University Press, 2011.

Lovibond, Sabrina. *Ethical Formation*. Cambridge, Massachusetts: Harvard University Press, 2002.

Macklin, Ruth. *Double Standards in Medical Research in Developing Countries*. Cambridge, UK: Cambridge University Press, 2004.

Mandal, Ananya. "History of Thalidomide," *News Medical*. http://www.news-medical.net/health/History-of-Thalidomide.aspx.

Marietta, Don. *For People and the Planet: Holism and Humanism in Environmental Ethics*, Philadelphia: Temple University Press, 1995.

Martensen, R. "The History of Bioethics: An Essay Review." Journal of the History of Medicine and Allied Sciences 56 no. 2 (2001a): 168–175.

Martensen, Robert. "The History of Bioethics: An Essay Review." Journal of the History of Medicine and Allied Sciences 56 no. 2 (2001b): 168–175.

Matolino, Bernard. 2011. "The (Mal) function of 'It' in Ifeanyi Menkiti's Normative Account of Person." African Studies Quarterly 12 no. 4 (2011): 25.

Mbiti, John. *African Religions and Philosophy*, New York: Praeger Publishers, 1970.

McNeil, Paul. "Research Ethics Review in Australia, Europe, and North America." IRB: Ethics and Human Research. The Hastings Center 11 no. 3 (1989): 4–7.

Meara, Naomi, Lyle Schmidt and Jeane Day. "Principles and Virtues: A Foundation for Ethical Decisions." The Counseling Psychologist 24 no. 1 (1996): 4–77. doi: 10.1177/0011000096241002.

Menkiti, Ifeanyi. "On the Normative Conception of a Person." In A Companion to African Philosophy, edited by Kwasi Wiredu, 324–331. Blackwell Publishing, 2004.

Menkiti, Ifeanyi. 1984. "Person and Community in African Traditional Thought." In African Philosophy, edited by R. Wright, 171–181. New York: University Press of America.

Merriam-Webster's Collegiate Dictionary. Eleventh Edition, Massachusetts: Merriam Webster, Inc., 2005.

Metz, Thaddeus. "Ikuenobe's Philosophical Perspectives on Communalism and Morality in African Traditions." Journal of Contemporary African Studies 26 no. 2 (2008): 231–239. doi:10.1080/03057240.2010.497618.

Myers, Linda. "Transpersonal Psychology: The Role of the Afrocentric Paradigm." Journal of Black Psychology 12 no. 1 (1985): 31–42.

Athanasoulis, Nafsika. "Virtue Ethics." *Internet Encyclopedia of Philosophy*: A Peer-reviewed Academic Resource, last modified April 09, 2014. http://www.iep.utm.edu/virtue/.

National Bioethics Advisory Commission. "Ethical and Policy Issues in Research Involving Human Participants." Report and Recommendations of the National Bioethics Commission, 1, Bethesda: Maryland, 2001.

Niehaus, I. "Bodies, Heat, and Taboos: Conceptualizing Modern Personhood in the South African Lowveld." Ethnology 41 no. 3 (2002): 189–207.

Nightingale, Stuart. "The Food and Drug Administration's Role in the Protection of Human Subjects." IRB: Ethics and Human Research, The Hastings Center 5 no. 1 (1983): 6–9.

Okere, Theophilus. Philosophy, Culture, and Society in Africa, Afro-Orbis Publications Ltd., Nsukka, Nigeria, 2005.

Okolo, Batholomew. "Self as a Problem in African Philosophy: Metaphysical Thinking in Africa." In Philosophy from Africa, edited by P. Coetzee and A. Roux. Oxford University Press, 2002.

Olin, John. "Community Preparedness for HIV Vaccine Trials in the Democratic Republic of Congo." Culture, Health & Sexuality 8 no. 6 (2006): 529–544.

Onywuenyi, Innocent. 1991. "Is There an African Philosophy?" In African Philosophy: The Essential Readings, edited by Tsenay Serequeberhan, 29–46. St. Paul: Paragon House, 1991.

Onyewuenyi, Innocent. *The African Origin of Greek Philosophy: An Exercise in Afrocentrism*. Nsukka: University of Nigeria Press, 2005.

Owomoyela, Oyeka. "Africa and the Imperative of Philosophy: A Skeptical Consideration." In African Philosophy: The Essential Readings, edited by Tsenay Serequeberhan, 29–46. St. Paul: Paragon House, 1991.

"Oath of Hippocrates." *Hippocratic Writings*. Translated by J.C. Chadwick and W.N. Man, 1950.

Palmer, Eric. "Corporate Responsibility and Freedom: A New Argument." In 7th IDEA International Conference Proceedings in Ethics and International Development on Accountability, Responsibility, and Integrity in Development: The Ethical Challenges in Sub-Saharan Africa and Beyond: From 19th–22nd July 2006, edited by Byaruhanga Rukooko. Makerere University, Kampala, Uganda, 2010.

Pellegrino, Edmund. 1999. "The Origins and Evolution of Bioethics: Some Personal Reflections." Kennedy Institute of Ethics Journal 9 no.1 (1999): 73–88.

Petryna, Adriana. *When Experiments Travel*, Princeton University Press, New Jersey, 2009.

Pierce, Jessica and Andrew Jameton. *The Ethics of Environmentally Responsible Health Care*, Oxford: Oxford University Press, Inc., 2004.

Piot, Charles. *Remotely Global: Village Modernity in West Africa*. Chicago, 1999.

Potter, Van. *Bioethics: Bridge to the Future*. Englewood Cliffs, New Jersey: Prentice-Hall, Inc., 1971.

Potter, Van. *Global Bioethics: Building on the Leopold Legacy*. East Lansing Michigan: Michigan State University Press, 1988.

Potter, Van. "Getting to the Year 3000: Can Global Bioethics Overcome Evolution's Fatal Flaw?" Perspectives in Biology and Medicine 34 no. 1 (1990): 89–98.

Potter, Van and Lisa Potter. 1995. "Forum: Global Bioethics: Converting Sustainable Development to Global Survival." Medicine and Global Survival 2 no. 3 (1995): 185–191.

Porter, Van Rensselaer and Peter Whitehouse. "Deep and Global Bioethics for a Livable Third Millennium." The Scientist, 12 (1998): 1–5.

Porter, Van and Peter Whitehouse. "Fragmented Ethics and 'Bridges Bioethics.'" Hastings Center Report 29, no. 1 (1999): 38–40.

Quigley, Dianne. "A Review of Improved Ethical Practices in Environmental and Public Health Research: Case Examples from Native Communities." Health Educational Behavior 33 no. 2 (2006): 130–147. doi: 10.1177/1090198104272053.

Raffoul, François. *The Origins of Responsibility*. Indianapolis: Indiana University Press, 2010.

Rehnquist, Janet. "The Globalization of Clinical Trials: A Growing Challenge in Protecting Human Subjects." U.S. Department of Health and Human Services, Office of Inspector General, Inspector General report, 2001.

Rendtorff, Jacob. "Basic Ethical Principles in European Bioethics and Biolaw: Autonomy, Dignity, Integrity and Vulnerability – Towards a Foundation of Bioethics and Biolaw." Medicine, Health Care and Philosophy 5 (2002): 235–244. doi:10.1023/A:1021132602330.

Riesman, Paul. "The Person and the Life Cycle in African Social Life and Thought." African Studies Review 29 no. 2 (1986): 71–138.

Risser, David. "Collective Moral Responsibility." (Other information missing), 2009.

Roberts, Paul. *The Impulse Society: America in the Age of Instant Gratification*. New York: Bloomsbury, 2014.

Roberts, Paul. "The Impulse Society." *Wellread*, TVW Television. http://www.tvw.org/index.php?option=com_tvwplayer&eventID=2015020019.

Robin, D. "Toward an Applied Meaning for Ethics in Business." Journal of Business Ethics 89 (2009): 139–150. doi: 10.1007/s10551-008-9990-y.

Roper, James. "*The Covenant of Democracy: Should Government be Run Like a Business?*" US: Kendall Hunt Publishing Company, 2012.

Rothman, David. *Strangers at the Bedside: A History of How Law and Bioethics Transformed Medical Decision Making*. New York: Aldine de Gruyter, 2003.

Ryan, Maura. 2004. Beyond a Western Bioethics? Theological Studies 65 no. 1 (2004): 158–177. doi: 10.1177/004056390406500105.

Schane, Sanford. "The Corporation as a Person: The Language of a Legal Fiction." Tulane Law Review, 61 (1986–87): 563–610.

Scheman, Naomi. "Narrative, Complexity, and Context: Autonomy as an Epistemic Value." In Naturalized Bioethics: Toward Responsible Knowing and Practice, edited by Hilde Lindermann, Marian Verkerk and Margaret Walker, 106–124. Cambridge: Cambridge University Press, 2009.

Schwartz, Shalom. Individualism-Collectivism: Critique and Proposed Refinements. Journal of Cross-Cultural Psychology 21 (1990): 139–157.

Schwartz, Shalom and Wolfgang Bilsky. "Towards a Theory of the Universal Content and Structure of Values: Extensions and Cross-Cultural Replications." Journal of Personality and Social Psychology 58 no. 5 (1990): 878–891.

Self, Lois. "Rhetoric and 'Phronēsis': The Aristotelian Ideal." Paper presented at the Annual Meeting of the Central States Speech Association. Chicago, 1978.

Senghor, Leopold. *On African Socialism*. New York: Stanford University Press, 1965.

Serequeberhan, Tsenay. *African Philosophy*. Minnesota: Paragon House, 1991.

Shaver, Kelly and Deborah Schutte. "Towards a Broader Psychological Foundation for Responsibility: Who, What, How." In Responsibility: The Many Faces of a Social Phenomenon, edited by Ann Auhagen and Hans-Werner Bierhoff, 35–48. London: Routledge, 2001.

Shapiro, Sydney. 1978. "Divorcing Profit Motivation from New Drug Research: A Consideration of Proposals to Provide the FDA with Reliable Test Data." Duke Law Journal, Ninth Annual Administrative Law Issue 155 (1978): 155–183.

Sladikas, Milto and Doris Schroeder. "Too Early for Global Ethics?" Cambridge Quarterly of Healthcare Ethics 14 (2005): 404–415.

Sosa, Ernest. *Knowledge in Perspective*. Cambridge: Cambridge University Press, 1991.

Sosa, Ernest. *A Virtue Epistemology*. Oxford: Clarendon Press, 2007.

Stanford Encyclopedia of Philosophy. "Virtue Ethics," modified on November 12, 2017. http://plato.stanford.edu/entries/ethics-virtue/.

Tangwa, Godfrey. "Some African Reflections on Biomedical and Environmental Ethics." In A Companion to African Philosophy, edited by Kwasi Wiredu, 387–395. Massachusetts: Blackwell Publishing Ltd., 2004a. doi: 10.1002/9780470997154.ch31.

Tangwa, Godfrey. "The Traditional African Perception of a Person: Some Implications for Bioethics." The Hastings Center Report 30 no. 5 (2000): 39–43.

Tempels, Placide. *Bantu Philosophy*. Preśence Africaine, 1959.

The White House Office of the Press Secretary. "Apology for Study Done in Tuskegee." May 16, 1997. http://clinton4.nara.gov/New/Remarks/Fri/19970516-898.html.

Trianosky, Gregory. "What is Virtue Ethics All About?" American Philosophical Quarterly 27 (1990): 335–344.

U.S. Government Printing Office. "Trials of War Crime before the Nuremberg Military Tribunals under Control Council." Washington 2 no. 10 (1949): 181–182.

U.S. Holocaust Memorial Museum. "Special Focus: The Doctors Trial: The Medical Case of the Subsequent Nuremberg Proceedings." http://www.ushmm.org/information/exhibitions/online-features/special-focus/doctors-trial.

U.S. National Institutes of Health. "Trends, Charts, and Maps." http://clinicaltrials.gov/ct2/resources/trends#RegisteredStudiesOverTimePostedResults.

U.S. Holocaust Memorial Museum. "The Doctors Trial: The Medical Case of the Subsequent Nuremberg Proceedings." http://www.ushmm.org/information/exhibitions/online-features/special-focus/doctors-trial.

Verharen, Charles. "Philosophy against Empire: An Ancient Egyptian Renaissance." Journal of Black Studies 36 no. 6 (2006): 958–973.

Verhoef, Heidi and Claudine Michel. "Studying Morality Within the African Context: A Model of Moral Analysis and Construction." Journal of Moral Education 26 no. 4 (1997): 389–407.

Well Read, http://www.tvw.org/index.php?option=com_tvwplayer&eventID=20150 20019. Accessed on February 5, 2015.

White, James. *Contemporary Moral Problems*. St. Paul: West Publishing Company, 1985.

Whitehouse, Peter. "The Ecomedical Disconnection Syndrome." The Hastings Center Report 29 no. 1 (1999): 41–44.

Widdows, Heather. "Is Global Ethics Moral Neo-colonialism? An Investigation of the Issue in the Context of Bioethics." Bioethics 21 no. 6 (2007): 305–315.

Wiredu, Kwasi. "Introduction: African Philosophy in Our Time." In A Companion to African Philosophy, edited by Kwasi Wiredu, 1–28. Blackwell Publishing, 2004.

World Health Organization, "Factsheet on the World Malaria Report 2013." http://www.who.int/malaria/media/world_malaria_report_2013/en/.

World Health Organization, "Dengue/Dengue Hemorrhagic Fever," http://www.who.int/csr/disease/dengue/en/.

World Health Organization. "Guidance Framework for Testing of Genetically Modified Mosquitoes." A Health Information Product by the WHO-executed UNICEF/UNDP/World Bank/World Health Organizations Special Program for Research and Training in Tropical Diseases, 2014.

World Health Organization: International Agency for Research on Cancer. Press Release no. 221, 2013.

World Medical Association. "Modern Physicians' Pledge Approved by World Medical Association." October 14, 2017. https://www.wma.net/news-post/modern-physicians-pledge-approved-by-world-medical-association/.

Zagzebski, Linda. *Virtues of the Mind: An Inquiry into the Nature of Virtue and Ethical Foundations of Knowledge*. Oxford: Clarendon Press, 1996.

Ziman, John. 1998. "Why Must Scientists Become More Ethically Sensitive than They Used to be?" Essays on Science and Society, Science 282 no. 5395 (1998): 1813–1814. doi: 10.1126/science.282.5395.1813.

Zimmerman, Michael. "Sharing Responsibility." American Philosophical Quarterly 22 no. 2 (1985): 115–122.

Additional/Recommended Literature

Ajayi, O. "Taboos and Clinical Research in West Africa." Journal of Medical Ethics 6 (1980): 61–63.

Ajuwon, Ademola and Nancy Kass. "Outcome of a Research Ethics Training Workshop Among Clinicians and Scientists in a Nigerian University." BMC Medical Ethics, 9 (2008): 1–9. doi:10.1186/1472-6939-9-1.

Dingwall, Robert and Vienna Rozelle. "The Ethical Governance of German Physicians, 1890–1939: Are There Lessons from History?" The Journal of Policy History 23 no. 1 (2011): 29–52. doi:10.1017/S0898030610000308.

Dubois, William. "New Drug Research, the Extraterritorial Application of FDA Regulations and the Need for International Cooperation." Vanderbilt Journal of Transnational Law 36 no. 161 (2003): 162–207.

Ezekwonna, Chukwuagozie. "African Communitarian Ethic: The Basis for the Moral Conscience and Autonomy of the Individual: Igbo Culture as a Case Study." *Theology* 809 (2005).

Metz, Thaddeus. "African and Western Moral Theories in a Bioethical Context." Developing World Bioethics, 10 no. 1 (2010): 49–58.

Metz, Thaddeus. "African Conceptions of Human Dignity: Vitality and Community as the Ground of Human Rights." in *Human Rights Review*, 13 (2012a): 19–37.

Metz, Thaddeus. 2012b. "An African Theory of Moral Status: A Relational Alternative to Individualism and Holism." Ethical Theory Moral Practice 15 (2012): 387–402.

Metz, Thaddeus. "Ethics in Africa and in Aristotle: Some Points of Contrast." Phronimon 13 no. 2 (2012c): 99–117.

Metz, Thaddeus. "The Motivation for 'Toward an African Moral Theory.'" South African Journal of Philosophy 26 no. 4 (2007a): 331–335.

Metz, Thaddeus. "Toward an African Moral Theory." The Journal of Political Philosophy 15 no. 3 (2007b): 321–341.

"National Code of Health Research Ethics," National Health Ethics Research Committee of Nigeria, Department of Health Planning and Research, Federal Ministry of Health, Abuja, Nigeria, 2006.

Ogunbanjo, G. and Knapp van Bogaert. "Communitarianism and Communitarian Bioethics." South African Family Practice 47 no. 10 (2005): 51–53.

Ojomo, A. "Environmental Ethics: An African Understanding." The Journal of Pan African Studies l4, no.3 (2011): 101–113.

WHO. "Biosafety for Human Health and the Environment in the Context of the Potential use of Genetically Modified Mosquitoes (GMMS): A Tool for Biosafety Training Based on Courses in Africa, Asia and Latin America, 2008–2011." Training Manual, 2016.

Omotonomila, Ikotun. "Legal Analysis of Globalization and Bioethics in Nigeria: In Depth Analysis of the Effect of Globalization on Bioethical Issues in a Third World Country and Proposed Legal Reforms to Protect the Polity." An unpublished document, 2004.

Onyemelukwe, Cheluchi. "Regulating Research Involving Humans in Nigeria: Some Recent Improvements." Health Law Review 16 no. 4 (2008): 36–46.

Tangwa, Godfrey. "Third Party-assisted Conception: An African Perspective." Theories of Medical Bioethics 29 (2008): 297–306.

Tangwa, Godfrey. "How Not to Compare Western Scientific Medicine with African Traditional Medicine." Developing World Bioethics 7 no. 1 (2007): 41–44.

Tangwa, Godfrey. 2004b. "Bioethics, Biotechnology and Culture: A Voice from the Margins." Developing World Bioethics 4 no. 2 (2004): 125–138.

Tangwa, Godfrey. "Bioethics: An African Perspective." Bioethics 10 no. 3 (1996): 183–200.

Tangwa, Godfrey. *Elements of African Bioethics in a Western Frame.* Cameroon: Langaa Research & Publishing Common Initiative Group, 2010.

Index

www.ingramcontent.com/pod-product-compliance
Lightning Source LLC
Chambersburg PA
CBHW071343230926
51846CB00002B/433